AYURVEDIC CLINIC SUCCESS BLUEPRINT

STEP BY STEP GUIDE TO ESTABLISHING AND GROWING YOUR PRACTICE

Dr Mukesh Aggarwal

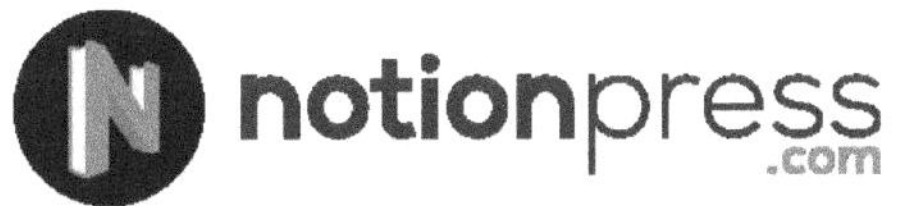

CONTENTS

PREFACE

Welcome to the journey of establishing and nurturing an Ayurvedic practice! This blueprint is a culmination of years of experience, dedication, and a deep-rooted passion for holistic healing. Ayurveda, an ancient science, holds timeless wisdom that resonates even more profoundly in today's fast-paced world.

In these pages strategies, and practical advice to guide aspiring practitioners and seasoned healers alike. The aim is not merely to create clinics but to foster sanctuaries of well-being, harmonizing traditional principles with modern healthcare needs.

The world of Ayurveda beckons with its holistic approach, offering a tapestry of possibilities for healing and wellness. This book is your companion, offering a roadmap from conceptualizing your clinic space to navigating the ever-evolving landscape of healthcare.

Each chapter encapsulates a vital aspect of crafting and nurturing an Ayurvedic practice. From designing an authentic clinic space to embracing technological innovations while preserving ancient wisdom, this guide aims to be a beacon, illuminating your path towards establishing a thriving Ayurveda practice.

May this blueprint inspire and empower you in your journey of blending ancient healing with contemporary care, ultimately fostering a future where Ayurveda thrives as a cornerstone of holistic well-being.

With warm regards,
Dr. Mukesh Aggarwal

ACKNOWLEDGMENTS

This endeavor would not have been possible without the support, guidance, and contributions of numerous individuals and entities. To all those who have lent their expertise, unwavering encouragement, and valuable insights, I extend my heartfelt gratitude.

I express deep appreciation to the pioneers of Ayurveda whose timeless wisdom continues to shape and inspire practitioners worldwide. Your dedication to preserving this ancient knowledge has paved the way for its continued relevance in modern healthcare.

I extend my gratitude to my mentors, colleagues, and friends in the Ayurvedic community whose shared wisdom and camaraderie have been invaluable in shaping this comprehensive guide. Your commitment to advancing Ayurveda is truly commendable.

A special acknowledgment goes to the patients who have entrusted us with their well-being. Your experiences and feedback have been instrumental in shaping the practices outlined in this blueprint.

I would also like to express my thanks to the publishers, editors, designers, and all those involved in bringing this book to fruition. Your dedication and expertise have transformed concepts into a tangible resource.

Lastly, to my family, whose unwavering support and understanding have been the cornerstone of this journey, I am forever grateful.

With profound appreciation,
Dr. Mukesh Aggarwal

INTRODUCTION TO AYURVEDA

<table>
<tr><td align="center">HIGHLIGHTS</td></tr>
<tr><td>

- Ayurveda, rooted in ancient wisdom, embodies a holistic approach to health, focusing on personalized, preventive care through balance and natural healing.
- Holistic healing principles underscore the interconnectedness of body, mind, and spirit, emphasizing individualized, preventive approaches for optimal well-being.

</td></tr>
</table>

UNDERSTANDING THE ESSENCE OF AYURVEDA

Ayurveda, originating from ancient India, encapsulates a profound understanding of holistic health and well-being.

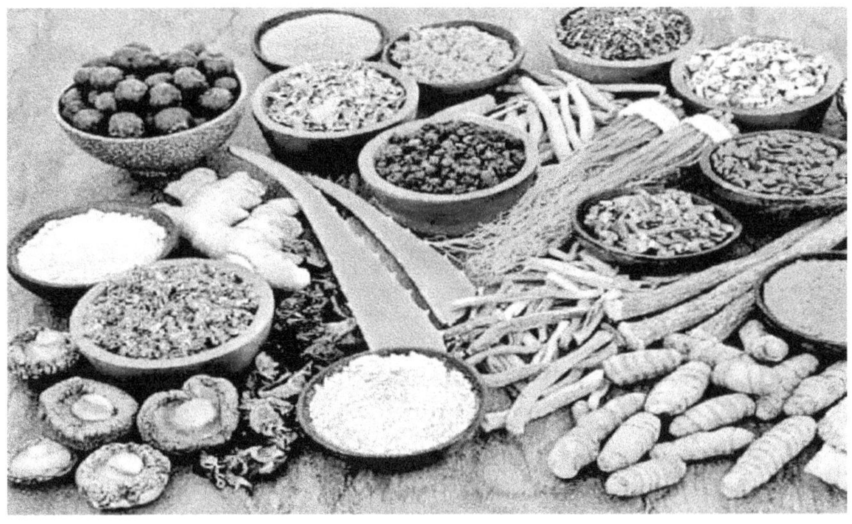

It embodies a philosophy that harmonizes the body, mind, and spirit, emphasizing balance and natural healing.

At its core, Ayurveda recognizes that each individual is unique, comprised of a distinct combination of the three doshas: Vata, Pitta, and Kapha. These doshas govern various bodily functions and, when in balance, promote health. Ayurvedic practitioners assess an individual's constitution and seek to restore balance through personalized treatments, which often involve herbal remedies, dietary adjustments, yoga, meditation, and lifestyle modifications.

Ayurveda's essence lies in its preventive approach, aiming to maintain health rather than merely treating diseases. It acknowledges the interconnectedness of an individual with their environment, emphasizing the importance of a harmonious relationship with nature. Seasonal routines, proper diet, and mindful living are key elements in Ayurvedic practices.

The holistic nature of Ayurveda extends beyond physical health, addressing mental, emotional, and spiritual well-being. It acknowledges the impact of emotions, stress, and mental states on one's health, promoting techniques to cultivate inner balance and resilience.

In today's world, where modern medicine often focuses on treating symptoms, Ayurveda stands as a beacon, offering a comprehensive understanding of health that transcends the mere absence of disease. Its timeless wisdom continues to inspire individuals seeking a balanced and harmonious life, bridging ancient traditions with contemporary wellness practices.

HOLISTIC HEALING PRINCIPLES

Holistic healing embodies a comprehensive approach to health, recognizing the interconnectedness of the body, mind, and spirit.

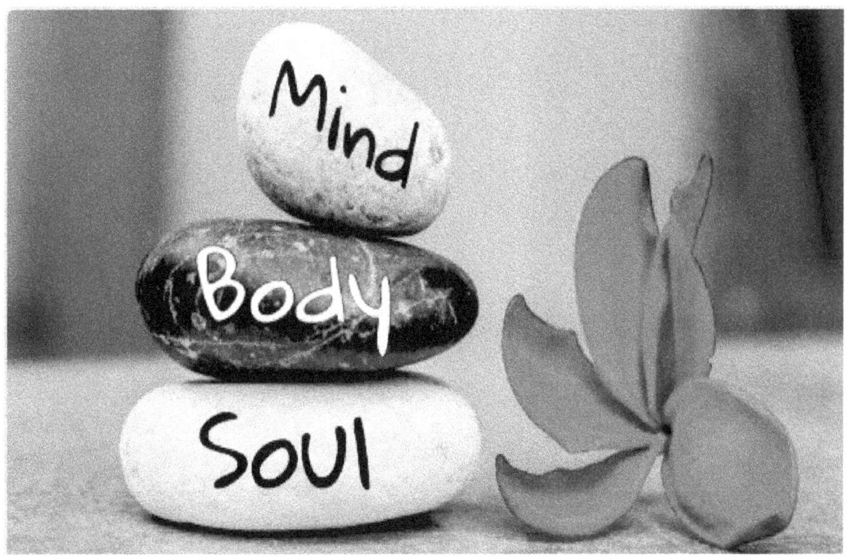

It embraces the understanding that an individual's well-being is influenced by various factors beyond physical symptoms, including emotional, mental, social, and spiritual aspects.

At its core, holistic healing emphasizes the body's innate ability to heal itself when provided with the right conditions. Rather than

solely focusing on alleviating symptoms, it seeks to address the root causes of illness, considering the entire person rather than isolated parts.

One fundamental principle of holistic healing is treating the person as a whole. This involves recognizing that physical ailments might have underlying emotional, mental, or spiritual origins. By exploring these interconnected aspects, holistic practitioners aim to restore balance and promote healing on multiple levels.

Another principle is the belief in individuality. Each person is unique, with their own set of experiences, genetics, environment, and lifestyle. Holistic healing takes into account these individual differences, tailoring treatments and approaches to meet each person's specific needs.

Prevention is also a cornerstone of holistic healing. Rather than waiting for illness to manifest, the focus is on maintaining wellness through lifestyle modifications, stress reduction techniques, proper nutrition, exercise, and practices that support mental and emotional balance.

Furthermore, holistic healing emphasizes the importance of the mind-body connection. It acknowledges the influence of thoughts, emotions, beliefs, and attitudes on physical health. Techniques such as meditation, mindfulness, and various forms of therapy are employed to foster a positive mental state, which can contribute to overall well-being.

Spirituality, in a non-religious sense, is often integrated into holistic healing principles. It involves connecting with a sense of purpose, meaning, and inner peace, recognizing the impact of spiritual well-being on one's health.

Overall, holistic healing principles advocate for a comprehensive, integrative approach that honors the complexity of the human being. By addressing all aspects of a person's life, it aims to promote not just the absence of disease, but a state of optimal health, vitality, and balance.

RELEVANCE OF AYURVEDA IN MODERN HEALTHCARE

Ayurveda's relevance in modern healthcare is gaining recognition due to its holistic approach, personalized treatments, and focus on preventive health measures. In the contemporary medical landscape, where there's a growing emphasis on integrative and personalized medicine, Ayurveda offers several elements that contribute significantly to healthcare:

Holistic Approach: Ayurveda considers the whole person—body, mind, and spirit. This aligns with the modern understanding of health that acknowledges the interconnectedness of various aspects of well-being. Integrating Ayurvedic principles can complement conventional treatments by addressing lifestyle factors, mental health, and emotional balance.

Personalized Medicine: Ayurveda's emphasis on individual constitution (doshas) and the unique balance of energies in each person allows for personalized treatments. In an era of precision medicine, this personalized approach is gaining traction as it tailors therapies, diets, and lifestyle recommendations to suit an individual's specific needs.

Preventive Health Measures: Ayurveda places great emphasis on preventive health strategies. By promoting a balanced lifestyle, dietary recommendations, seasonal routines, and stress reduction techniques, it aligns with the modern healthcare focus on preventing diseases rather than just treating them.

Natural and Holistic Therapies: Ayurvedic treatments often involve the use of natural herbs, dietary modifications, yoga, meditation, and detoxification practices. These non-invasive and holistic therapies are increasingly sought after as alternatives or complements to conventional medical interventions.

Mind-Body Connection: Ayurveda recognizes the intricate relationship between mental health and physical well-being, which modern medicine is also increasingly acknowledging. Techniques within Ayurveda, such as mindfulness, meditation, and yoga, can contribute to managing stress, anxiety, and improving overall mental health.

Global Interest and Research: With growing interest worldwide,

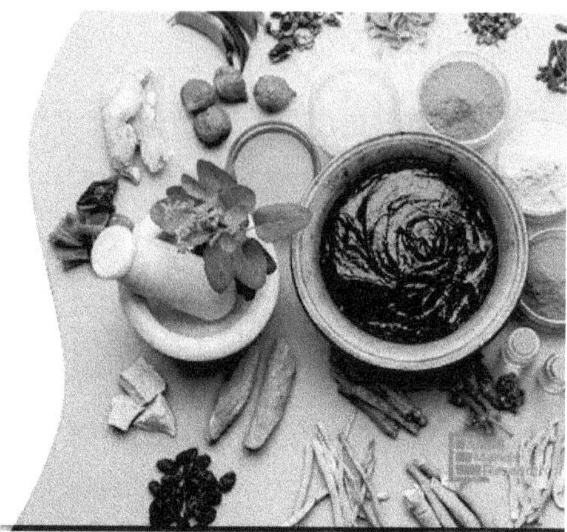

scientific research is exploring the efficacy and safety of Ayurvedic practices. Integrating evidence-based Ayurvedic therapies into modern healthcare systems could offer more comprehensive and diverse treatment options.

Chapter 2

SETTING UP YOUR AYURVEDIC CLINIC

HIGHLIGHTS
The key message encapsulates two main facets: the art of creating an authentic Ayurvedic space that embodies balance and nature, coupled with the essential considerations for legally establishing a clinic equipped to provide holistic healing in adherence to regulations.

DESIGNING AN AUTHENTIC AYURVEDIC SPACE

Designing an authentic Ayurvedic space is a nuanced art, blending ancient wisdom with modern aesthetics. Ayurveda, rooted in harmony and balance, guides the creation of such spaces. From the outset, a deep understanding of Ayurvedic principles and their manifestation in architecture, colors, textures, and elements is essential.

The foundation rests upon the five elements (Pancha Mahabhutas) – earth, water, fire, air, and space. Incorporating these elements through materials like natural woods, stones, flowing water features, fire pits, and ample open spaces aligns the design with Ayurvedic philosophies.

The space's layout must facilitate the flow of energy (Prana). Ensuring proper ventilation, allowing natural light to fill the space, and integrating elements that promote tranquility and relaxation support this energy flow. Zones for different Ayurvedic practices like yoga, meditation, or massage should harmoniously coexist within the space.

Color plays a pivotal role in influencing energies and moods. Warm, earthy tones resonate with Ayurvedic principles, while vibrant accents can represent the three doshas (Vata, Pitta, Kapha) – reflecting their balance within the environment.

Furnishings and decor must prioritize natural, organic materials. Furniture shapes and textures should embrace simplicity and comfort, facilitating relaxation and balance. Art and ornamentation, inspired by nature, can evoke a sense of connection with the universe, enhancing the holistic experience.

Incorporating aromatic herbs, essential oils, and incense aligns with Ayurvedic practices, stimulating the senses and fostering healing. Thoughtful placement of plants and greenery not only purifies the air but also establishes a connection with nature, a fundamental aspect of Ayurveda.

Lastly, creating a serene ambiance involves sound and space utilization. Soft, calming music or sounds of nature can deepen the holistic experience. The space should encourage a sense of mindfulness and contemplation.

In essence, designing an authentic Ayurvedic space involves a holistic approach, considering physical, mental, and spiritual aspects. It's a symphony of ancient wisdom, modern design sensibilities, and a deep reverence for the interconnectedness of humans and nature.

ESSENTIAL EQUIPMENT AND SUPPLIES FOR AYURVEDIC CLINIC

Outfitting an Ayurvedic clinic involves careful consideration of specialized equipment and supplies essential for providing holistic healing and wellness services rooted in Ayurvedic principles.

Treatment Tables: Specialized tables designed for various treatments

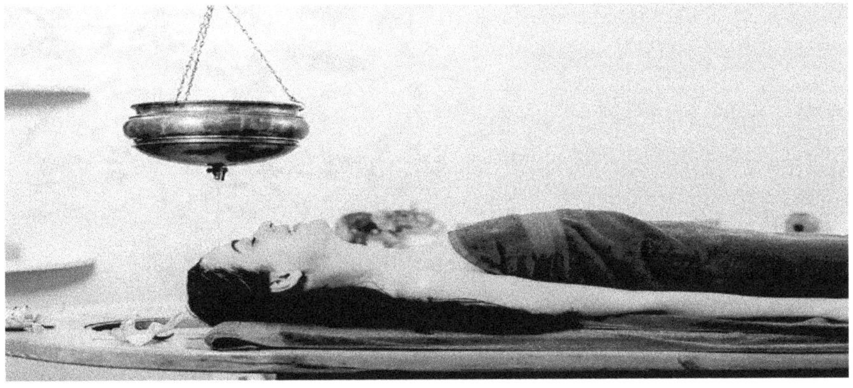

like Abhyanga (oil massage) or Shirodhara (oil pouring) are fundamental. They should be sturdy, comfortable, and adjustable to accommodate different procedures.

Steam Cabinets or Steam Boxes: Integral for Swedana (herbal steam therapy) to induce sweating and detoxification. These cabinets maintain the temperature and humidity required for the therapy.

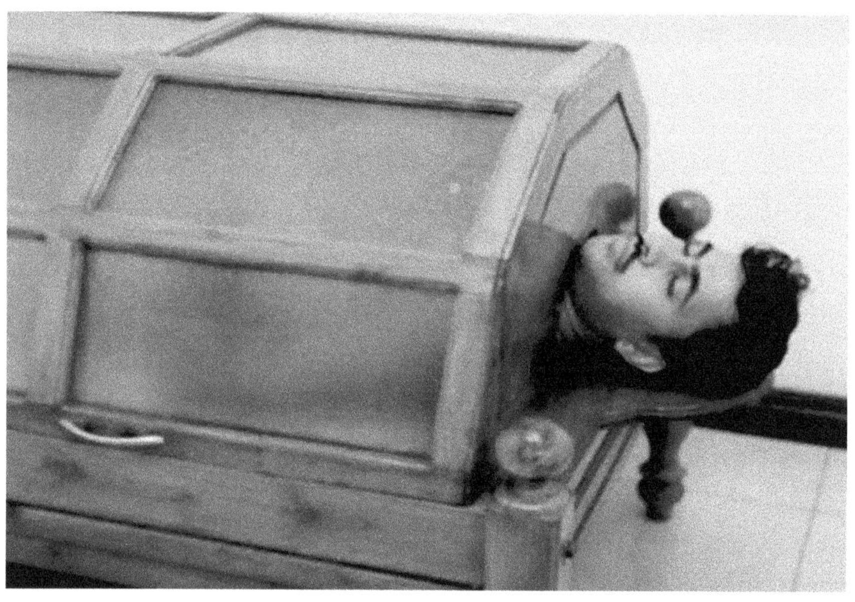

Herbs and Herbal Preparations: A wide array of Ayurvedic herbs, oils, powders, and medicated ghee for preparing customized treatments based on individual doshas and ailments.

Ayurvedic Oils and Massage Tools: High-quality oils such as sesame, coconut, or herbal-infused oils for therapies. Tools like Kansa wands or rollers aid in specific massages.

Copper Vessels and Utensils: Used for preparing herbal decoctions, storing water, or serving therapeutic drinks. Copper is believed to have healing properties in Ayurveda.

Tongue Cleaners and Neti Pots: Essential for daily cleansing practices like tongue scraping and nasal irrigation (Neti) to maintain oral and nasal hygiene.

Incense, Essential Oils, and Aromatherapy Supplies: Used to create a soothing ambiance and stimulate the senses during treatments and therapies.

Yoga Props and Meditation Cushions: Supporting clients in practicing yoga or meditation enhances the holistic approach to healing.

Diagnostic Tools: Including Nadi Pariksha (pulse diagnosis) tools and other assessment instruments to determine a person's dosha imbalance and overall health status.

Educational Materials: Books, charts, or digital resources that educate clients about Ayurvedic principles, doshas, diet, and lifestyle.

Sanitization and Hygiene Supplies: Proper disinfectants, cleaning supplies, and disposable linens to maintain cleanliness and hygiene.

Consultation and Documentation Tools: Software or systems to manage client records, track treatments, and schedule appointments efficiently.

Each piece of equipment and supply plays a crucial role in delivering authentic Ayurvedic therapies and services. The integration of these elements ensures a conducive environment for healing and promotes the balance of mind, body, and spirit in individuals seeking Ayurvedic care.

LEGALITIES, PERMITS, AND REGULATIONS FOR ESTABLISHING AN AYURVEDIC CLINIC

Establishing an Ayurvedic clinic involves navigating various legalities, permits, and regulations to ensure compliance with local, national, and sometimes international standards for healthcare facilities and holistic practices.

Licensing and Accreditation: Obtaining the necessary licenses from local health authorities or regulatory bodies is crucial. This might involve specific certifications or accreditations that validate the clinic's adherence to safety, hygiene, and quality standards.

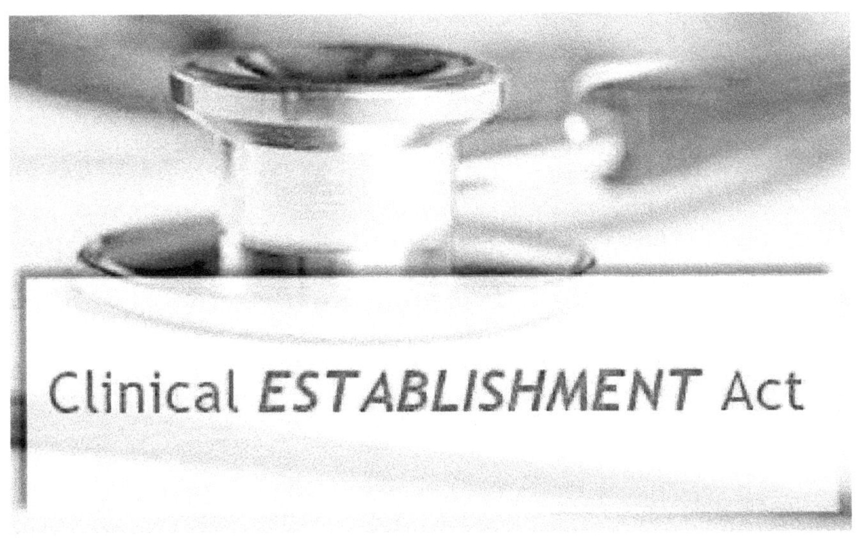

Business Registration: Registering the clinic as a legal entity, such as a sole proprietorship, partnership, or corporation, is essential. This involves obtaining a business license and fulfilling tax obligations in accordance with local laws.

Zoning and Building Permits: Ensuring the clinic location complies with zoning regulations and obtaining building permits for renovations or construction is necessary. Certain areas might have specific zoning requirements for healthcare facilities.

Healthcare Compliance and Standards: Following healthcare regulations and standards applicable to clinics and holistic healthcare practices is crucial. This includes maintaining patient confidentiality, adhering to sanitation and safety protocols, and meeting healthcare service standards.

Practitioner Licensing and Qualifications: Ensuring that practitioners employed or associated with the clinic possess the required licenses, certifications, and qualifications to practice Ayurveda or other holistic therapies is imperative.

Drug and Herb Regulations: Adhering to regulations governing the use, storage, and dispensing of herbs, oils, and Ayurvedic medicines is crucial. Some jurisdictions have strict guidelines regarding the sourcing and distribution of herbal products.

Advertising and Marketing Regulations: Following advertising and marketing guidelines specific to healthcare services is essential. This might include restrictions on claims made about treatments or services provided by the clinic.

Insurance and Liability Coverage: Obtaining appropriate insurance coverage, including liability insurance for practitioners and the clinic itself, helps mitigate risks associated with healthcare services.

International Regulations (if applicable): If the clinic plans to offer services to international clients or import/export herbal products, understanding and complying with international regulations and trade laws becomes essential.

Continuing Education and Professional Development: Staying updated with evolving regulations, industry standards, and advancements in Ayurvedic practices through ongoing education and professional development is beneficial for ensuring compliance and maintaining high-quality care.

Navigating these legalities, permits, and regulations demands meticulous planning, consultation with legal experts, and a thorough understanding of both healthcare and business laws. Compliance ensures the clinic operates ethically, safely, and efficiently while providing authentic Ayurvedic care to patients within the boundaries of the law.

Chapter 3

CRAFTING YOUR UNIQUE PRACTICE

HIGHLIGHTS
Define your Ayurveda clinic's niche by understanding your strengths, market demands, unique offerings, and ideal clientele.
Build an Ayurvedic brand rooted in holistic principles, authenticity, client-centric care, and community engagement while crafting tailored treatment plans based on individual assessments and Ayurvedic principles.

DEFINE YOUR AYURVEDA CLINIC NICHE

Defining your Ayurveda clinic's niche involves a strategic process:

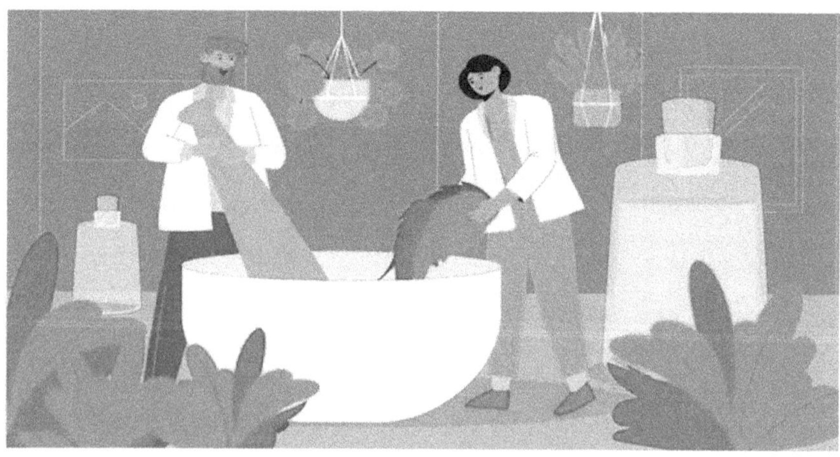

Self-Assessment: Identify your strengths, passions, and experti
se within Ayurveda.

What treatments or aspects of Ayurveda are you most skilled and passionate about?

Market Research: Analyze the local or broader market to understand the needs and gaps in Ayurvedic services. Look for unmet demands or specific health concerns prevalent in your area.

Identify Unique Offerings: Pinpoint what makes your clinic unique. It could be specialized treatments, personalized care, unique herbal formulations, or a particular focus such as stress management, chronic illnesses, fertility, or rejuvenation.

Target Audience: Define your ideal clientele. Consider demographics, lifestyle preferences, health concerns, and cultural inclinations. Tailor your offerings to cater specifically to their needs and preferences.

Competitor Analysis: Assess other Ayurvedic clinics in your area. Identify their strengths and weaknesses to carve out your distinct position. Find an angle that differentiates your clinic from others.

Brand Narrative: Craft a compelling story that communicates your clinic's values, philosophy, unique offerings, and how your specialization benefits your clients.

Client Feedback and Adaptation: Collect feedback from initial clients and adjust your offerings based on their experiences and suggestions. Continuously refine and adapt your niche to better serve your clientele.

Consistency and Quality: Ensure consistency in delivering high-quality services aligned with your identified niche. Establish a reputation for excellence within your chosen specialization.

Marketing Strategy: Develop a marketing plan that targets your specific niche audience. Utilize online platforms, networking, collaborations, and word-of-mouth to reach and engage with your potential clients.

Continuous Improvement: Stay updated with advancements in Ayurveda, integrate new research, and incorporate innovative techniques to enhance your clinic's offerings.

Defining your clinic's niche requires a balance between your expertise, market demands, and client needs. Regularly reassess and adapt to stay relevant and competitive in the Ayurvedic healthcare space.

BUILD A BRAND THAT REFLECTS AYURVEDIC VALUES

Building a brand that embodies Ayurvedic values involves a thoughtful process aligned with the core principles of Ayurveda. Here are steps to help create a brand reflective of these values:

1. Embrace Ayurvedic Principles:

Holistic Approach: Emphasize holistic wellness, considering mental, physical, and spiritual health in your brand ethos.

Balance and Harmony: Highlight the importance of balance and harmony in life through your brand messaging. Natural and Organic: Promote the use of natural, organic ingredients in your products or treatments, aligning with Ayurvedic principles.

2. Define Your Brand's Purpose:

Establish a clear mission and vision that aligns with Ayurvedic principles of promoting health, longevity, and well-being.

Communicate how your brand contributes to the greater good of individuals' health and wellness in a holistic manner.

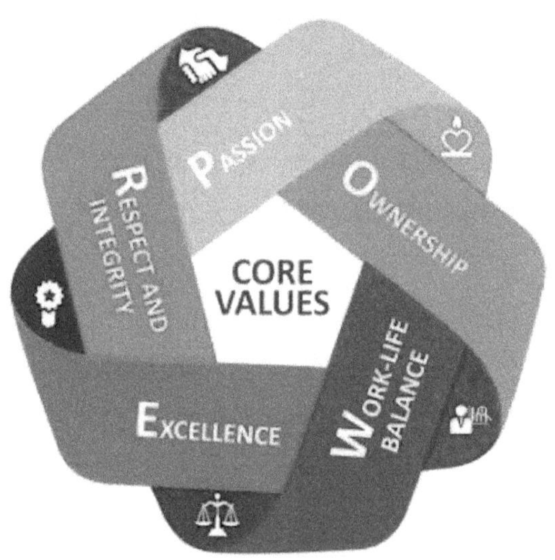

3. Authenticity and Transparency:

Be transparent about your practices, ingredients, and treatment methodologies. Authenticity is key in building trust with your audience.

Share the stories behind your brand, your journey, and the philosophy that drives your Ayurvedic clinic.

4. Visual Identity:

Use natural, earthy colors and imagery that reflect the essence of Ayurveda.

Incorporate symbols or elements associated with Ayurveda in your logo, packaging, and marketing materials to establish recognition.

5. Educational Content:

Educate your audience about Ayurveda through blogs, workshops, or social media content. Share valuable insights, tips, and information about Ayurvedic practices and their benefits.

6. Client-Centric Approach:

Put the client's well-being at the forefront. Offer personalized experiences, attentive care, and a nurturing environment aligned with Ayurvedic principles.

7. Ethical Business Practices:

Uphold ethical practices in sourcing ingredients, manufacturing, and providing services. Show commitment to sustainability, fair trade, and eco-friendliness.

8. Consistency and Integration:

Ensure that all aspects of your clinic – from services and products to staff interactions and customer service – consistently reflect Ayurvedic values.

9. Engage with the Community:

Engage in community events, wellness programs, or collaborations that promote Ayurvedic values and contribute to community well-being.

Building a brand rooted in Ayurvedic values requires a deep understanding and integration of these principles across all aspects of your clinic's operations, communications, and client interactions. Consistency and authenticity will help in creating a brand that resonates with individuals seeking Ayurvedic wellness solutions.

DEVELOP TAILORED TREATMENT PLANS FOR YOUR AYURVEDIC CLINIC

Developing tailored treatment plans in an Ayurvedic clinic involves a personalized approach based on individual health assessments and Ayurvedic principles. Here's a guide:

1. Initial Consultation:

Conduct a comprehensive assessment of the client's health, including medical history, lifestyle, diet, emotional well-being, and any specific health concerns.

2. Prakriti Analysis:

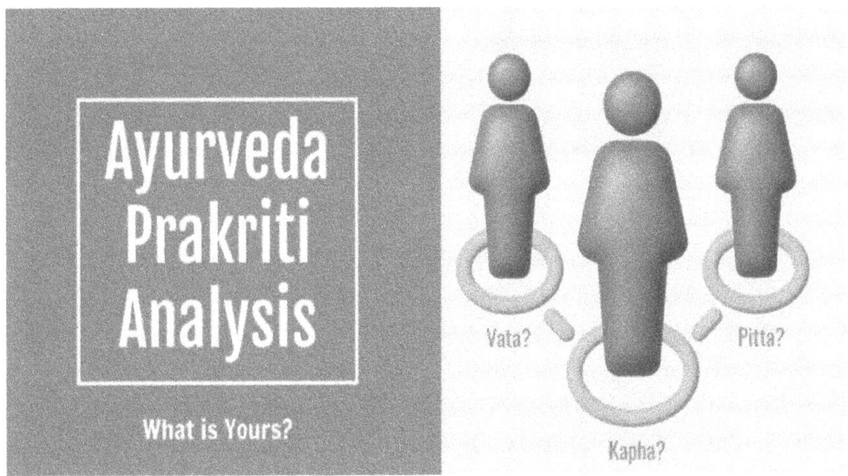

Determine the client's Prakriti (unique constitutional type) through thorough examination, which involves assessing their dominant doshas (Vata, Pitta, Kapha).

3. Vikriti Assessment:

Evaluate the imbalance (Vikriti) in doshas, identifying any deviations from their natural state that contribute to health issues.

4. Treatment Customization:

Based on the Prakriti and Vikriti assessment, tailor treatment plans incorporating personalized recommendations in diet, lifestyle modifications, herbal remedies, and therapies.

5. Lifestyle Modifications:

Suggest lifestyle adjustments aligned with Ayurvedic principles, such as incorporating specific yoga poses, meditation, exercise routines, sleep patterns, and stress management techniques.

6. Dietary Recommendations:

Prescribe a personalized diet plan considering the client's Prakriti and Vikriti. Recommend specific foods, spices, and eating habits to restore balance and address health issues.

7. Herbal Remedies and Supplements:

Recommend Ayurvedic herbs, supplements, or formulations to support the body's natural healing processes, targeting specific imbalances or health concerns.

8. Therapies and Treatments:

Create a customized treatment regimen including Panchakarma (detoxification), Abhyanga (oil massage), Shirodhara (oil treatment for the head), or other therapies tailored to address the client's needs.

9. Regular Follow-ups and Adjustments:

Schedule follow-up sessions to monitor progress and make necessary adjustments to the treatment plan based on the client's response and changes in their health.

10. Holistic Approach:

Emphasize the holistic nature of Ayurveda by addressing not only physical symptoms but also mental and emotional well-being.

11. Education and Empowerment:

Educate clients about Ayurvedic principles, their body constitution, and lifestyle practices to empower them to take an active role in their well-being.

12. Collaboration and Communication:

Encourage open communication between practitioners and clients, and consider collaborating with other healthcare professionals to provide comprehensive care.

Tailoring treatment plans in Ayurveda involves a personalized, holistic approach that addresses the unique constitution and health concerns of each individual, focusing on restoring balance and promoting overall well-being.

NURTURING PATIENTS RELATIONSHIPS

<table>
<tr><td align="center">HIGHLIGHTS</td></tr>
<tr><td>Effective healthcare hinges on empathetic communication, trust-building, and personalized care tailored to individual needs, fostering engagement and optimizing patient outcomes.</td></tr>
</table>

EFFECTIVE COMMUNICATION AND CONSULTATION TECHNIQUES

Effective communication and consultation techniques

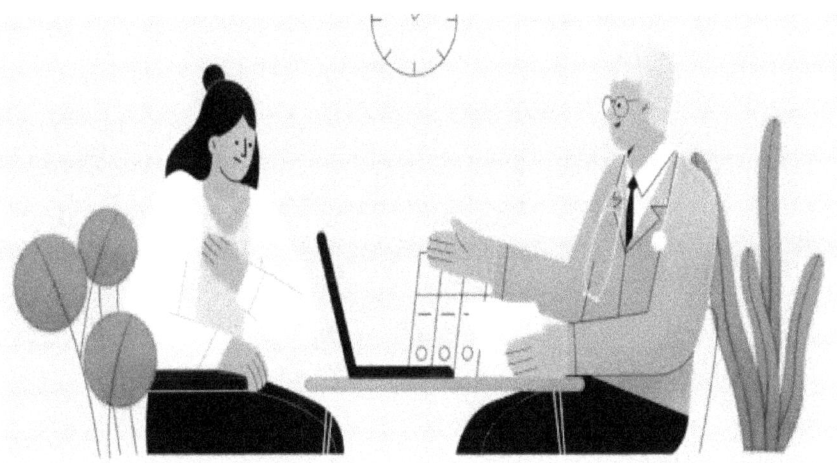

play a pivotal role in the healthcare sector, particularly between healthcare professionals and patients.

The ability to communicate clearly, listen actively, and engage empathetically greatly influences patient satisfaction, understanding of medical information, adherence to treatment plans, and overall health outcomes.

Active Listening: Firstly, establishing rapport through attentive listening is fundamental. Active listening involves not just hearing what the patient says, but also understanding their concerns, emotions, and unspoken cues. This forms the foundation for a trusting relationship, where patients feel valued, respected, and heard. Moreover, effective communication involves the use of clear and simple language to convey complex medical information, ensuring patients comprehend their diagnosis, treatment options, and potential risks.

Empathy: employing empathy in communication is essential. Understanding a patient's emotional state and acknowledging their feelings fosters a supportive environment. Empathetic communication helps alleviate anxiety, builds confidence, and encourages patients to share pertinent information crucial for accurate diagnosis and treatment planning.

Non Verbal Cues: In addition to verbal communication, non-verbal cues such as body language, eye contact, and gestures significantly impact patient interactions. Maintaining open body language and appropriate eye contact conveys attentiveness and sincerity, while gestures can aid in illustrating medical concepts or procedures, enhancing patient understanding.

Shared Decision-Making: Effective consultation techniques involve shared decision-making. Engaging patients in discussions about their treatment options, involving them in decision-making processes, and considering their preferences and values empower patients to actively participate in their healthcare journey. This collaborative approach often leads to improved adherence to treatment plans and better health outcomes.

Cultural Competence: Another crucial aspect of effective communication is cultural competence. Understanding and respecting diverse cultural backgrounds, beliefs, and values are essential in ensuring effective communication and avoiding misunderstandings or misinterpretations that can impact patient care.

To conclude, effective communication and consultation techniques are indispensable in healthcare. They not only facilitate the exchange of information but also nurture a patient-centric approach, promoting trust, understanding, and better health outcomes. Healthcare professionals equipped with these skills contribute significantly to enhanced patient satisfaction, compliance, and overall quality of care.

CULTIVATING TRUST AND RAPPORT WITH PATIENTS

In the realm of healthcare, cultivating trust and rapport between healthcare providers and patients is indispensable. This foundational relationship serves as the bedrock upon which effective communication, successful treatment outcomes, and patient satisfaction are built.

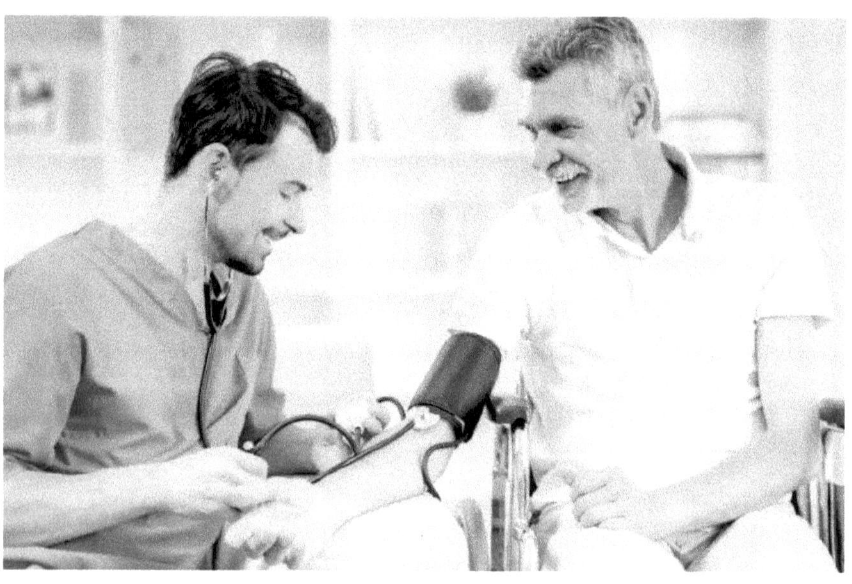

Firstly, trust is a cornerstone in healthcare interactions. Patients entrust their well-being, health information, and often their lives to healthcare professionals. Establishing trust involves demonstrating competence, integrity, and empathy. Healthcare providers who exhibit expertise and professionalism instill confidence in patients, assuring them that their care is in capable hands.

Moreover, empathy and active listening play pivotal roles in fostering rapport. Empathizing with a patient's concerns, fears, and emotions creates a sense of connection. When healthcare providers actively listen to patients, they convey respect, understanding, and genuine interest, laying the groundwork for a trusting relationship. Patients who feel heard and understood are more likely to disclose crucial information, adhere to treatment plans, and actively engage in their healthcare journey.

Transparency is another vital aspect of cultivating trust. Openly discussing diagnoses, treatment options, and potential risks promotes transparency. When healthcare providers engage in honest and clear communication, patients are better equipped to make informed decisions about their care. Transparency also involves acknowledging limitations or uncertainties, which further reinforces trust by demonstrating humility and honesty.

Consistency and reliability are key elements in nurturing trust over time. Consistent behavior, timely responses, and reliable care contribute to a patient's confidence in their healthcare team. Whether it's promptness in scheduling appointments or delivering accurate information, reliability strengthens the patient-provider relationship.

Additionally, building rapport encompasses respecting patients' autonomy and involving them in decision-making. Respecting their preferences, values, and individual circumstances empowers patients and fosters a sense of partnership in their healthcare journey. Collaborating with patients in setting goals and making informed choices strengthens the bond between healthcare providers and patients.

In conclusion, cultivating trust and rapport in healthcare is multifaceted. It involves a combination of competence, empathy, transparency, reliability, and respect for patient autonomy. By prioritizing these elements, healthcare providers can create an environment where patients feel valued, supported, and confident in their care, ultimately leading to improved patient satisfaction and better health outcomes.

PERSONALIZING EXPERIENCES FOR OPTIMAL HEALING

In the dynamic landscape of healthcare, the concept of personalized experiences has emerged as a pivotal element in promoting optimal healing and well-being among patients. Personalizing healthcare journeys involves tailoring treatments, communication, and overall care to meet the unique needs, preferences, and circumstances of each individual.

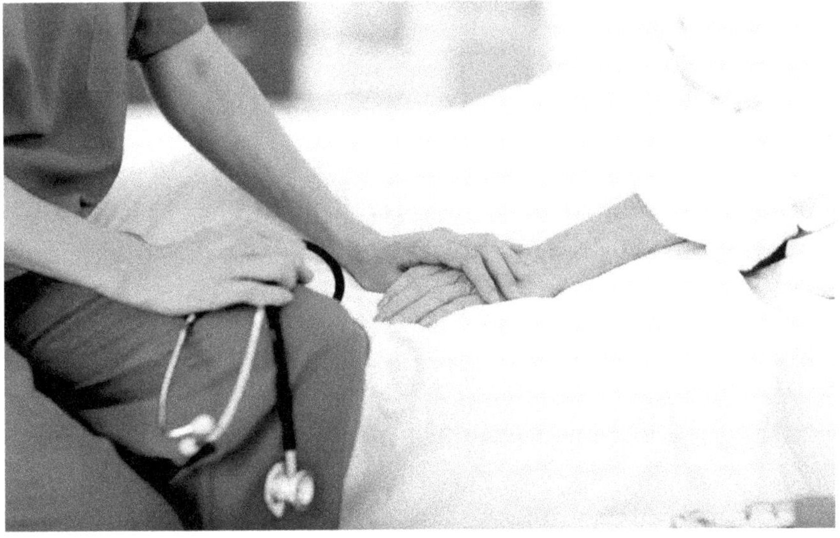

Firstly, personalized care acknowledges the diversity among patients. Every individual brings a distinct set of values, beliefs, cultural backgrounds, and health circumstances to their healthcare journey. Recognizing and respecting these differences allows healthcare providers to create tailored approaches that resonate with each patient, fostering a deeper connection and understanding.

Furthermore, personalizing experiences in healthcare involves a comprehensive understanding of patients' preferences. Acknowledging patient preferences—whether related to treatment options, communication styles, or care settings—empowers individuals to actively engage in their health management. When patients feel their preferences are considered, they become more invested in their care, leading to improved adherence and better health outcomes.

Additionally, personalized care emphasizes the importance of communication. Effectively communicating medical information in a manner that aligns with the patient's level of understanding and using language that resonates with their background and experiences is crucial. This approach not only ensures comprehension but also promotes trust and a sense of partnership between healthcare providers and patients.

Personalized experiences extend beyond medical treatment to encompass emotional support and holistic well-being. Recognizing the emotional aspects of illness, addressing fears and anxieties, and providing empathetic support contribute significantly to the healing process. A personalized approach attends not only to the physical ailment but also to the emotional and psychological needs of patients, fostering a sense of care and compassion integral to healing.

Moreover, leveraging technology in healthcare allows for further personalization. Tailoring treatment plans, providing remote consultations, or utilizing wearable devices to monitor health parameters cater to individual needs and preferences, enhancing patient engagement and promoting a sense of ownership over one's health.

Chapter 5

MARKETING STRATEGIES FOR SUCCESS

HIGHLIGHTS
<ul><li>Marketing Strategies: Embrace digital tools, local collaborations, and patient-centric content to reach holistic health enthusiasts effectively.</li><li>Networking & Content Creation: Foster connections within the Ayurveda community, while creating patient-centric, clear, and engaging educational materials to build trust in holistic healthcare.</li></ul>

Marketing strategies for an Ayurvedic clinic can be diverse and effective in reaching a wider audience interested in holistic health practices. Here are several strategies:

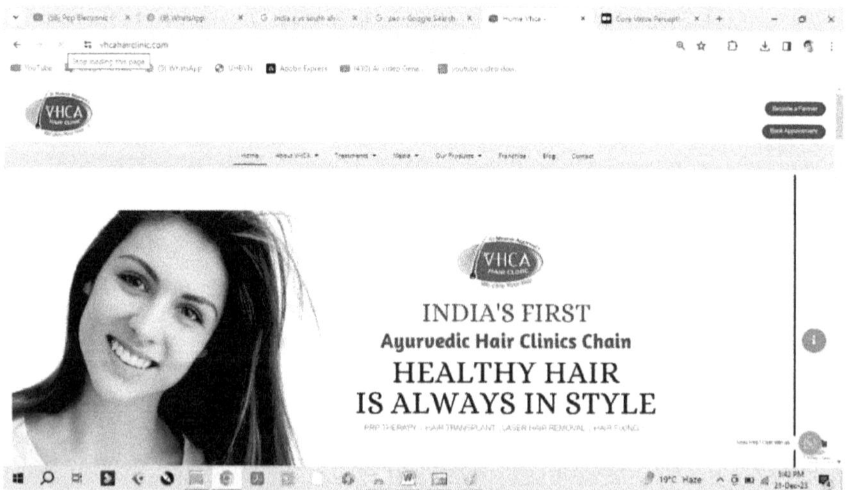

Professional Website: Develop an informative and visually appealing website showcasing the clinic's services, practitioners, treatments, and testimonials. Ensure it's user-friendly and optimized for mobile devices.

Search Engine Optimization (SEO): Implement SEO techniques to improve the clinic's visibility on search engines. Focus on keywords related to Ayurveda, holistic health, and local search terms to attract potential clients in the area.

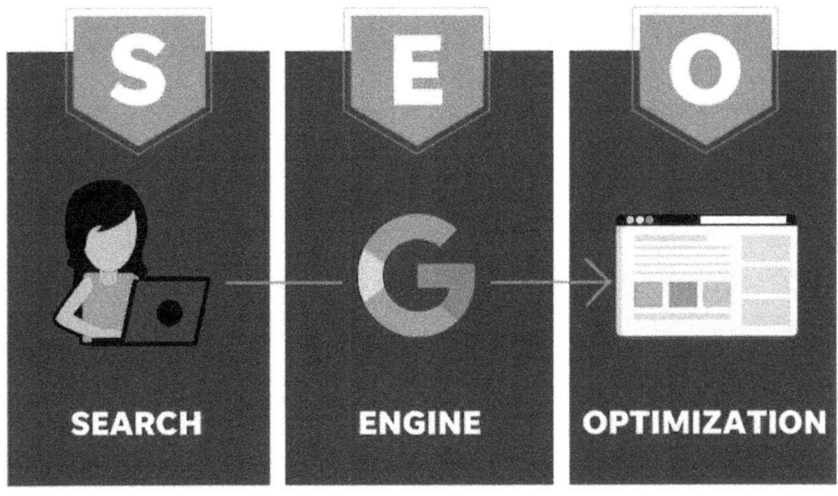

Content Marketing: Create high-quality content such as blog posts, articles, e-books, or videos covering topics related to Ayurveda, wellness tips, herbal remedies, etc. Share these on the website and social media platforms to engage and educate the audience.

Social Media Presence: Leverage platforms like Instagram, Facebook, and YouTube to share educational content, success stories, patient testimonials, and updates about the clinic. Engage with the audience by responding to comments and messages.

Email Marketing: Implement an email campaign to send newsletters, promotions, health tips, and updates about the clinic's services. Personalize content to cater to the specific interests of subscribers.

Local Partnerships and Events: Collaborate with local wellness centers, gyms, spas, or yoga studios for cross-promotions or joint events. Participate in health fairs, workshops, or community events to raise awareness about the clinic.

Online Advertising: Utilize targeted online ads on platforms like Google Ads or social media to reach a specific demographic interested in holistic health and Ayurveda. Consider retargeting campaigns to engage with previous website visitors.

Patient Referral Program: Encourage satisfied patients to refer friends and family by offering incentives or discounts for referrals. Word-of-mouth referrals can be powerful in attracting new clients.

Free Workshops or Webinars: Host free educational sessions on Ayurveda, wellness practices, or specific health topics relevant to the audience. This helps showcase expertise and builds trust among attendees.

Online Booking and Teleconsultation: Simplify the appointment booking process by offering online scheduling and teleconsultation services, making it convenient for clients to access the clinic's services.

Remember, consistency and measurement are crucial. Continuously assess the effectiveness of these strategies through analytics and adapt based on what works best for the clinic's goals and target audience.

NETWORKING WITHIN THE AYURVEDA COMMUNITY

Networking within the Ayurveda community is an invaluable asset for Ayurvedic doctors, fostering collaboration, knowledge sharing, and professional growth. In a field deeply rooted in tradition and holistic healing, establishing connections with peers, experts, and organizations can significantly benefit an Ayurveda doctor's practice and career.

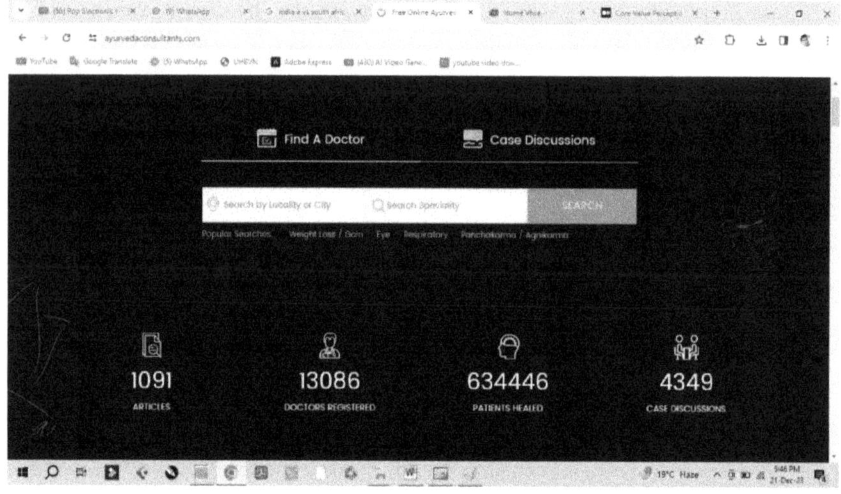

Firstly, networking offers opportunities for continuous learning and skill enhancement. Engaging with fellow Ayurvedic practitioners through seminars, conferences, or workshops enables the exchange of insights, new research, and diverse treatment approaches. This exposure to varying perspectives enriches an Ayurvedic doctor's expertise, keeping them updated with the latest advancements in the field.

Collaboration within the Ayurvedic community can lead to shared resources and expertise, potentially enhancing the quality of patient care. Building relationships with other Ayurveda doctors, herbalists, therapists, and wellness practitioners can facilitate referrals, allowing patients to access comprehensive and holistic healthcare services.

Moreover, networking provides a platform to showcase individual expertise and contribute to the broader Ayurvedic community. Sharing case studies, research findings, or unique treatment methodologies not only elevates an Ayurveda doctor's professional reputation but also contributes to the collective knowledge base of the community.

Participating actively in professional associations, online forums, or social groups dedicated to Ayurveda fosters a sense of belonging and support. These networks offer a space for discussions, mentorship opportunities, and guidance, creating a conducive environment for personal and professional development.

Establishing connections with suppliers of authentic Ayurvedic herbs, medicines, or wellness products is also crucial. A reliable network of suppliers ensures access to high-quality ingredients, maintaining the integrity of treatments and enhancing patient satisfaction.

Networking doesn't limit itself to professionals alone; connecting with patients, community leaders, and influencers interested in holistic healthcare can broaden the reach of an Ayurvedic doctor's practice. Engaging with these groups fosters trust, increases awareness, and attracts individuals seeking alternative and holistic healing solutions.

In conclusion, networking within the Ayurveda community is an essential component for the growth, knowledge enrichment, and collaboration opportunities for Ayurvedic doctors. Building strong connections, sharing expertise, and actively engaging with various stakeholders contribute not only to individual professional development but also to the advancement and promotion of Ayurveda as a holistic healthcare system.

CREATING COMPELLING CONTENT AND EDUCATIONAL MATERIALS FOR PATIENTS

Crafting compelling Ayurveda content and educational materials for patients is pivotal in fostering understanding, trust, and engagement with this holistic healthcare system. In a world where information is readily accessible, providing valuable and easily understandable content can empower patients to embrace Ayurveda principles and practices for their well-being.

To begin, personalized and informative content tailored to patients' needs and concerns is essential. This includes explaining fundamental Ayurvedic concepts, such as doshas (body constitutions), the importance of balanced lifestyle, dietary recommendations, and the holistic approach to wellness. Presenting this information in a clear, jargon-free manner helps patients grasp the essence of Ayurveda and its relevance to their health.

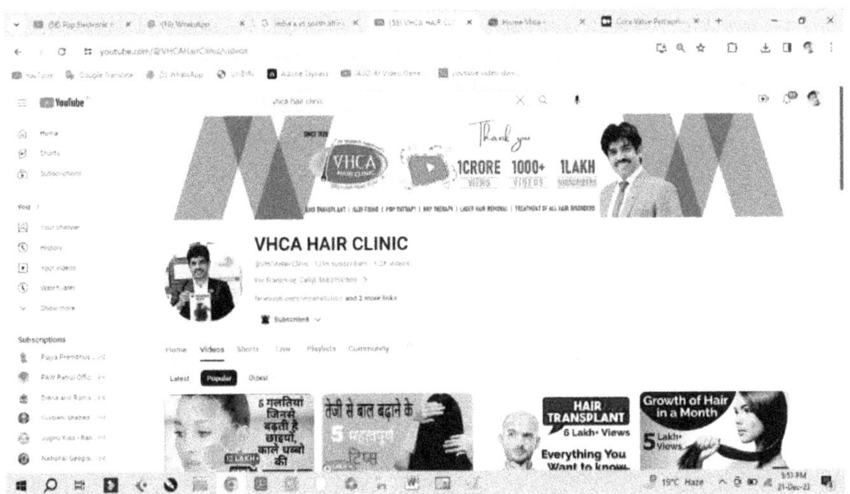

Visual aids, such as infographics, videos, or illustrated guides, can enhance the understanding of complex concepts. Incorporating visuals to explain concepts like Ayurvedic body types or illustrating Ayurvedic routines can make the information more accessible and memorable for patients.

Sharing real-life stories, testimonials, or case studies of individuals who have benefited from Ayurvedic treatments helps in establishing credibility and building trust. Personal narratives resonate deeply with patients, inspiring confidence and belief in the efficacy of Ayurveda.

Creating educational materials that address common health concerns or conditions, along with Ayurvedic perspectives and solutions, is invaluable. For instance, developing guides for managing stress, improving digestion, or enhancing sleep through Ayurvedic practices demonstrates the practical application of these ancient principles in everyday life.

Consistency in producing quality content across various platforms, including websites, social media, newsletters, and printed materials, ensures a continuous flow of educational resources for patients. Regularly updating and diversifying content keeps patients engaged and encourages them to explore and adopt Ayurveda as a holistic lifestyle choice.

Offering interactive elements like quizzes, self-assessment tools, or downloadable resources allows patients to actively engage with the content, aiding in self-discovery of their unique constitutions and health needs. These tools can guide patients towards personalized Ayurvedic recommendations and encourage active participation in their wellness journey.

Lastly, seeking patient feedback and being responsive to their queries or concerns creates a sense of inclusivity and encourages a dialogue. Addressing patient inquiries or misconceptions promptly reinforces trust and demonstrates the clinic's commitment to patient education and care.

In conclusion, creating compelling Ayurveda content and educational materials involves a patient-centric approach, clarity in communication, visual aids, relatable stories, practical guidance, interactive elements, and responsiveness. These efforts not only educate patients about Ayurveda but also inspire them to integrate its principles into their lives for holistic well-being.

Chapter 6

OPERATIONAL EFFICIENCY AND MANAGEMENT

HIGHLIGHTS
• Optimizing an Ayurvedic clinic involves efficient scheduling, standardized protocols, staff training, and technology integration, enhancing patient care and operational effectiveness. • Successful clinic management prioritizes competent staffing, ongoing training, effective team dynamics, and patient-centered care for holistic success.

STREAMLINING AYURVEDIC CLINIC OPERATIONS

Streamlining operations within an Ayurvedic clinic is essential for enhancing patient care, optimizing resources, and fostering overall efficiency. By implementing strategic measures, the clinic can effectively manage various aspects, from patient intake to treatment procedures and administrative tasks.

The initial step involves optimizing patient scheduling and intake processes. Implementing an efficient appointment system, either through digital platforms or specialized software, reduces waiting times and enhances patient satisfaction. Furthermore, digitizing patient records and histories ensures accessibility and streamlined information retrieval for practitioners, thereby expediting diagnosis and treatment planning.

Standardizing treatment protocols and procedures maintains consistency in care delivery. Establishing clear guidelines for therapies, prescriptions, and follow-ups enables practitioners to provide comprehensive and uniform treatment while ensuring patient safety and satisfaction.

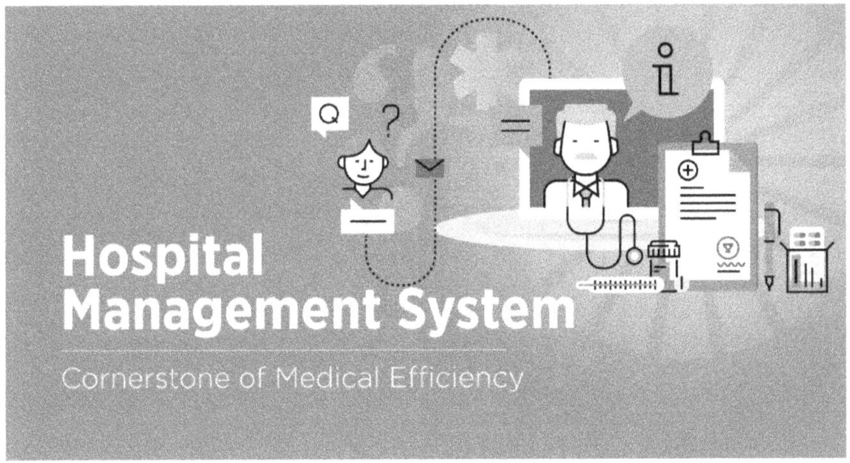

Efficient inventory management plays a pivotal role in an Ayurvedic clinic. Monitoring herbal medicines, oils, and other supplies ensures availability while preventing wastage or shortages. Implementing an inventory tracking system assists in maintaining optimal stock levels, reducing costs, and ensuring timely procurement.

Staff training and development programs are crucial for enhancing operational efficiency. Regular training sessions on updated practices, technological advancements, and customer service skills empower the staff to deliver high-quality care while adapting to changes within the field of Ayurveda.

Incorporating technology, such as telemedicine or online consultations, extends the clinic's reach beyond its physical location. This approach enables remote patient care, consultation, and follow-ups, offering convenience to patients while expanding the clinic's potential client base.

Streamlining administrative tasks, including billing, invoicing, and insurance processing contribute significantly to overall operational efficiency. Automated systems or dedicated personnel for administrative duties reduce errors, save time, and enhance the financial health of the clinic.

Lastly, seeking feedback from patients and staff fosters continuous improvement. Implementing suggestions and addressing concerns demonstrates the clinic's commitment to providing exceptional care and ensures that operational enhancements align with the needs of both patients and practitioners.

In conclusion, optimizing operations within an Ayurvedic clinic involves a multifaceted approach encompassing technology adoption, standardized procedures, staff training, and patient-centric care. Streamlining these aspects ensures enhanced patient experiences, improved clinical outcomes, and sustainable growth for the clinic.

AYURVEDIC CLINIC STAFFING, TRAINING AND TEAM MANAGEMENT

Creating a successful Ayurvedic clinic involves more than just treatment methodologies—it's about nurturing a competent and cohesive team. Staffing, training, and team management play pivotal roles in ensuring the clinic's effectiveness, patient satisfaction, and overall success.

Staffing begins with recruiting individuals who align with the clinic's values, possess relevant skills, and exhibit a passion for Ayurveda. Hiring practitioners well-versed in Ayurvedic principles, along with competent administrative and support staff, forms the foundation of a capable team.

Once assembled, ongoing training is essential to keep the team updated with the latest advancements in Ayurveda, ensuring they provide cutting-edge care. Regular work-shops, seminars, and training sessions not only enhance their knowledge but also foster a culture of continuous learning and improvement within the clinic.

Team management revolves around effective leadership, communication, and collaboration. A strong leader provides direction, support, and mentorship, fostering a positive work environment and encouraging professional growth among team members. Open communication channels and regular team meetings facilitate the exchange of ideas, addressing challenges, and fostering a sense of belonging and teamwork.

Ensuring a harmonious balance between the clinic's practitioners, administrative staff, and support personnel is crucial. Each role is integral to the clinic's smooth functioning, and acknowledging the significance of every team member's contributions encourages synergy and mutual respect.

Implementing performance evaluation systems helps identify strengths and areas for improvement among team members. Constructive feedback and recognition of achievements motivate staff and contribute to individual growth and overall team effectiveness.

Promoting a patient-centric approach is at the core of team management in an Ayurvedic clinic. Encouraging empathy, compassion, and personalized care among staff members cultivates strong patient relationships and enhances the clinic's reputation.

In summary, staffing, training, and team management are essential pillars in establishing and maintaining a successful Ayurvedic clinic. By recruiting skilled individuals, providing continuous training, fostering effective team dynamics, and prioritizing patient care, the clinic can achieve operational excellence and ensure a fulfilling experience for both patients and staff alike.

IMPLEMENTING EFFICIENT SCHEDULING AND BILLING SYSTEMS

Implementing efficient scheduling and billing systems is crucial for the smooth operation of any healthcare facility, including an Ayurvedic clinic. These systems not only enhance patient satisfaction but also streamline administrative processes, improving overall efficiency and revenue management.

Efficient scheduling systems are the backbone of a well-organized clinic. Implementing digital scheduling software or platforms allows for easy appointment booking, reducing wait times and optimizing the utilization of practitioners' time. Integrating features such as automated reminders and confirmations minimizes no-shows, ensuring a more consistent flow of patients.

Moreover, a well-designed scheduling system takes into account practitioner availability, treatment duration, and patient preferences. This ensures a balanced workload for practitioners and enhances patient convenience by offering suitable appointment slots.
Billing systems in an Ayurvedic clinic must be accurate, transparent, and user-friendly. Implementing electronic billing software streamlines the invoicing process, reducing errors and delays. It allows for efficient management of patient billing information, insurance claims, and payment tracking, ensuring timely reimbursements and improved cash flow.

Integration of billing systems with patient records and treatment data eliminates redundancies and errors, facilitating a seamless billing process. Furthermore, offering multiple payment options, including online payment gateways or installment plans, enhances patient convenience and satisfaction.

Training staff on utilizing these systems optimally is essential. Staff should be well-versed in navigating the scheduling and billing software, ensuring smooth operations and avoiding potential errors that could affect patient experience and financial stability.

Regular system audits and updates are crucial for maintaining the efficiency of scheduling and billing systems. Ensuring compliance with industry standards and adapting to technological advancements enhances the clinic's capabilities and keeps it aligned with best practices.

The implementation of efficient scheduling and billing systems in an Ayurvedic clinic not only streamlines operations but also contributes to improved patient experiences, reduced administrative burdens, and enhanced financial management. It ultimately allows the clinic to focus more on delivering quality care while maintaining a robust administrative framework.

Chapter 7

INTEGRATING TRADITIONAL WISDOM WITH MODERN SCIENCE

HIGHLIGHTS
Collaboration between Ayurvedic and modern medicine enhances patient care by merging ancient wisdom with modern science, fostering holistic well-being. Integrating diverse medical modalities offers a comprehensive approach, prioritizing prevention, and personalized treatments for improved health outcomes.

COLLABORATION WITH CONVENTIONAL MEDICINE PRACTITIONERS

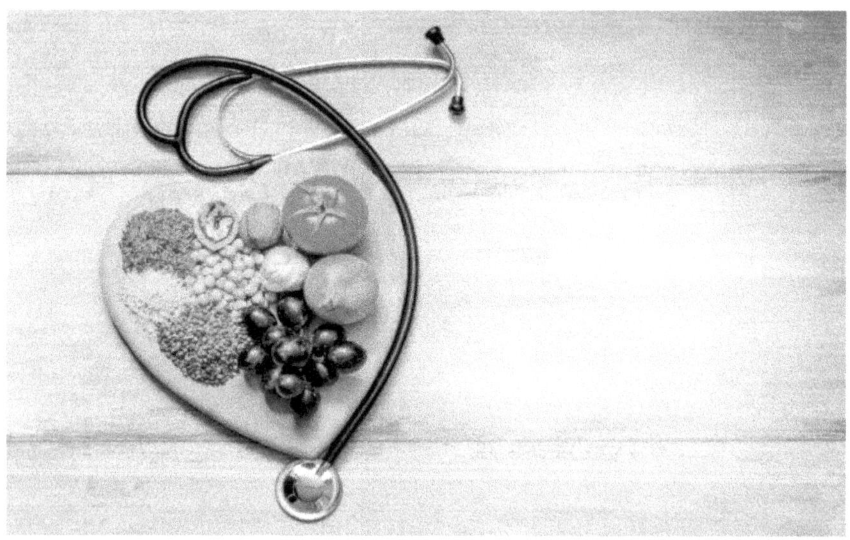

The collaboration between Ayurvedic practitioners and conventional medicine practitioners can bring holistic care to patients, merging traditional wisdom with modern science. This collaboration fosters a comprehensive approach to health, drawing on the strengths of both disciplines to enhance patient outcomes.

Ayurveda, rooted in ancient Indian knowledge, focuses on personalized treatments considering an individual's constitution and emphasizes natural remedies, lifestyle modifications, and dietary changes. On the other hand, conventional medicine relies on scientific research, advanced technologies, and pharmaceutical interventions to manage diseases.

When these two systems collaborate, patients can benefit from a wider range of treatment options. For instance, Ayurvedic practices like herbal remedies, yoga, and dietary adjustments can complement conventional treatments, potentially reducing side effects and improving overall well-being. Moreover, Ayurvedic practitioners can provide insights into preventive healthcare, promoting holistic lifestyle changes that complement conventional interventions.

Effective collaboration involves mutual respect, understanding, and open communication between practitioners. It requires sharing knowledge, experiences, and research findings to create integrated treatment plans tailored to each patient's needs. Regulatory frameworks that acknowledge and support this collaboration are also essential for its success.

In conclusion, the collaboration between Ayurvedic and conventional medicine practitioners holds tremendous potential in delivering patient-centered care that merges the best of both worlds, ultimately enhancing health outcomes and promoting wellness.

BRIDGING ANCIENT AYURVEDIC KNOWLEDGE WITH CONTEMPORARY RESEARCH

Bridging ancient Ayurvedic knowledge with contemporary research represents a powerful union of traditional wisdom and modern scientific exploration. This fusion offers a pathway to validate and integrate centuries-old Ayurvedic practices into today's evidence-based healthcare landscape.

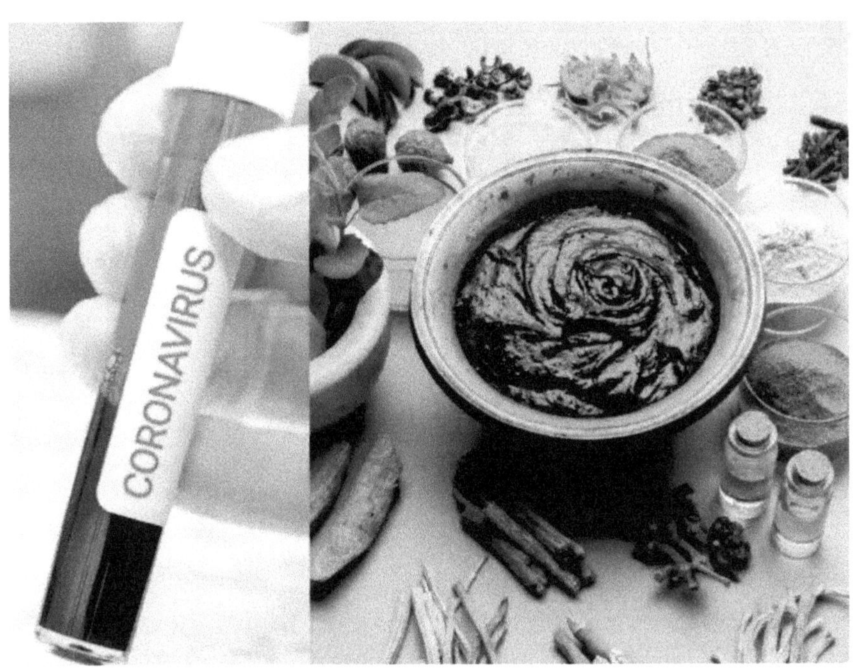

Ayurveda, steeped in ancient Indian traditions, emphasizes a holistic approach to health, considering an individual's mind, body, and spirit. It advocates personalized treatments, herbal remedies, dietary modifications, and lifestyle adjustments to restore balance and prevent illness. However, the lack of scientific validation has sometimes led to skepticism within the modern medical community.

Contemporary research techniques provide an opportunity to bridge this gap by subjecting Ayurvedic principles to rigorous scientific scrutiny. Through clinical trials, molecular studies, and other scientific methodologies, researchers can investigate the efficacy, safety, and mechanisms of action behind Ayurvedic practices.

By marrying ancient knowledge with modern scientific validation, several benefits emerge. Firstly, it allows for a deeper understanding of the mechanisms underlying Ayurvedic treatments, fostering greater acceptance and integration into mainstream healthcare. Secondly, validated Ayurvedic practices can complement conventional medicine, potentially offering alternative or adjunctive therapies with fewer side effects.

This bridge also supports the development of standardized protocols and guidelines, ensuring consistency and safety in the practice of Ayurveda. Moreover, it opens doors for collaborative research initiatives, where Ayurvedic principles and contemporary medical advancements converge to create innovative healthcare solutions.

Efforts to bridge Ayurvedic knowledge with contemporary research demand collaboration between Ayurvedic practitioners, scientists, and healthcare institutions. This collaboration facilitates the sharing of knowledge, methodologies, and resources, fostering a symbiotic relationship between ancient wisdom and modern science.

In conclusion, bridging ancient Ayurvedic knowledge with contemporary research holds immense promise in validating and integrating traditional practices into modern healthcare. This synergy not only preserves the rich heritage of Ayurveda but also offers opportunities for enhanced healthcare outcomes, paving the way for a more comprehensive and inclusive approach to well-being.

FOSTERING A BALANCED APPROACH TO HEALTHCARE

Fostering a balanced approach to healthcare involves embracing a comprehensive perspective that integrates various medical modalities, emphasizing both prevention and treatment while considering the individual's physical, mental, and emotional well-being.

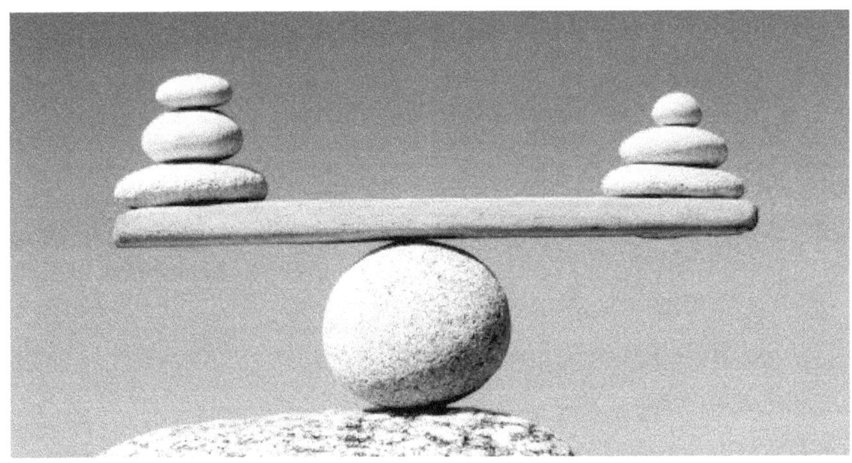

A balanced healthcare approach acknowledges the value of conventional medicine's advancements, including pharmaceuticals, surgeries, and technological innovations. It appreciates their efficacy in treating acute conditions and managing complex diseases. However, it also recognizes the limitations and potential side effects of these interventions, prompting the exploration of alternative or complementary approaches.

In this balanced model, holistic practices such as Ayurveda, Traditional Chinese Medicine, naturopathy, and mind-body therapies play a crucial role. These modalities focus on prevention, lifestyle modifications, natural remedies, and personalized treatments tailored to an individual's unique constitution.

The synergy between conventional medicine and holistic practices offers several advantages. Integrating these approaches allows for a more comprehensive understanding of health and disease. It encourages preventive measures and lifestyle changes that address root causes rather than merely managing symptoms. Additionally, it provides patients with a wider array of treatment options, promoting patient-centered care and empowering individuals to actively participate in their health journey.

The key to fostering this balanced approach lies in collaborative efforts among healthcare practitioners, researchers, policymakers, and patients. It requires open-mindedness, mutual respect, and effective communication between different medical paradigms. Furthermore, educational initiatives that emphasize the integration of diverse medical approaches and encourage interdisciplinary learning are essential.

Regulatory frameworks that support and accommodate this integration are also crucial. These frameworks should ensure patient safety, standardization of practices, and ethical considerations while allowing for the flexibility to incorporate diverse healthcare modalities.

In conclusion, fostering a balanced approach to healthcare involves embracing the strengths of both conventional medicine and holistic practices. By integrating various modalities and promoting preventive care alongside treatment, this approach aims to provide comprehensive, patient-centered healthcare that considers the individual's holistic well-being.

Chapter 8

NAVIGATING CHALLENGES AND GROWTH

HIGHLIGHTS
Addressing Ayurveda's hurdles involves integrating it with modern medicine, ensuring quality, education, research, global recognition, and accessibility. Sustainable clinic scaling means holistic services, personalized care, tech integration, community engagement, and financial stability. Continuing education empowers practitioners with evolving knowledge, skills, evidence-based practices, and ethical standards for optimal patient care and professional growth.

ADDRESSING COMMON OBSTACLES IN AYURVEDIC PRACTICE

Ayurveda, the ancient system of medicine rooted in the Indian subcontinent, faces several obstacles in its modern-day practice. While it offers holistic healing and personalized wellness, certain challenges impede its widespread adoption and implementation. Understanding and addressing these hurdles are crucial for harnessing Ayurveda's full potential.

Integration with Modern Medicine: One significant obstacle is the integration of Ayurveda with conventional medicine. Bridging the gap between these two systems requires collaborative efforts, acknowledgment of each system's strengths, and research to validate Ayurvedic practices within the framework of evidence-based medicine.

Standardization and Quality Control: Ayurvedic treatments often involve herbal remedies, oils, and therapies. However, inconsistent quality, lack of standardization, and adulteration of herbal products pose concerns about their efficacy and safety. Establishing robust quality control measures and standardized procedures is essential to ensure reliability and safety in Ayurvedic interventions.

Education and Training: The shortage of well-trained Ayurvedic practitioners is another obstacle. Comprehensive education, updated curriculum, and practical training are vital to produce competent professionals. Integrating Ayurvedic teachings into mainstream medical education can also enhance understanding and acceptance among healthcare providers.

Research and Evidence: Despite its long history, Ayurveda sometimes lacks empirical evidence to support its practices. Encouraging and funding research studies to validate Ayurvedic treatments, understand their mechanisms, and demonstrate their effectiveness is crucial for wider acceptance and incorporation into healthcare systems.

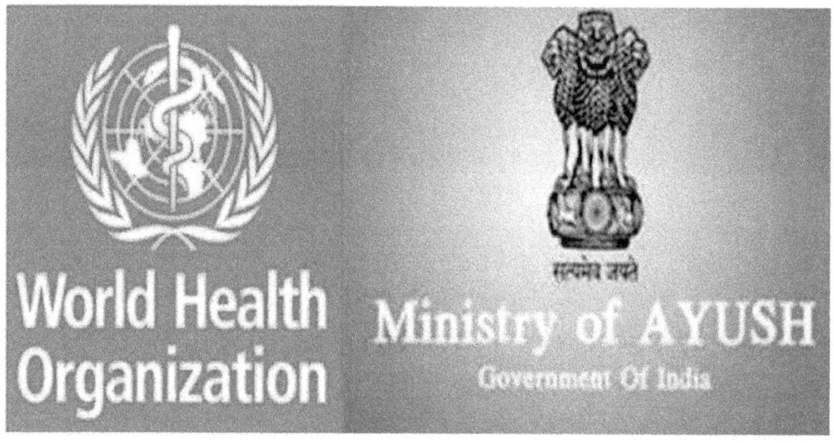

Global Recognition and Regulation: Ayurveda's global recognition faces challenges due to varying regulations and standards across countries. Developing international guidelines and regulations while respecting cultural differences can facilitate its recognition as a valid healthcare system worldwide.

Consumer Awareness and Accessibility: Enhancing awareness among the general population about Ayurveda's principles, benefits, and limitations is essential. Making Ayurvedic services accessible and affordable ensures broader adoption and acceptance.

Addressing these obstacles requires a multi-dimensional approach involving collaboration among practitioners, policymakers, researchers, and the public. By overcoming these challenges, Ayurveda can rightfully claim its place in providing holistic healthcare solutions in the modern world.

SCALING YOUR AYURVEDIC CLINIC SUSTAINABLY

As an Ayurvedic practitioner aiming to expand your clinic, sustainable scaling involves strategic planning and a holistic approach. Building upon the principles of Ayurveda itself, here's a blueprint for sustainable growth:

Holistic Service Expansion: Rather than merely increasing patient numbers, focus on offering a wider range of Ayurvedic services. Introduce specialized therapies, wellness programs, yoga sessions, and nutritional counseling. Ensure that each new service aligns with Ayurvedic principles and complements existing offerings.

Practitioner Development: Invest in continuous education for your staff. Encourage them to deepen their understanding of Ayurveda, explore advanced therapies, or specialize in specific areas. Well-trained practitioners enhance the clinic's reputation and attract more clients.

Personalized Patient Care: Maintain the core of Ayurveda—personalized care. Even with scaling, prioritize individual attention, tailoring treatments to each patient's unique constitution and health needs. This personalized approach fosters trust and loyalty among your clientele.

Technological Integration: Embrace technology to streamline operations while maintaining the human touch. Implement electronic health records, online appointment systems, and telemedicine for consultations. However, ensure that technology enhances rather than replaces the personal connection with patients.

Community Engagement and Education: Organize workshops, seminars, or community events to raise awareness about Ayurveda. Engaging with the community not only spreads knowledge but also fosters a sense of belonging and trust in your clinic's expertise.

Quality Assurance and Accreditation: Focus on maintaining high standards. Seek accreditation or certifications that validate your clinic's adherence to quality practices.

This not only builds credibility but also attracts a discerning clientele.

Financial Sustainability: Scale your clinic gradually while ensuring financial stability. Develop a sustainable business model that considers revenue streams, cost management, and reinvestment for growth. Avoid rapid expansion that strains resources and compromises service quality.

Collaboration and Networking: Foster relationships with other healthcare providers, both conventional and alternative. Collaborations can lead to referrals, knowledge exchange, and a more comprehensive approach to patient care.

Feedback and Adaptation: Regularly seek feedback from patients and staff. Adapt and evolve based on these inputs, ensuring that your clinic continues to meet the changing needs and expectations of your clientele.

By embracing sustainable scaling practices, your Ayurvedic clinic can grow organically without compromising the essence of Ayurveda—holistic, personalized care rooted in ancient wisdom. This approach ensures not just expansion, but also the preservation of the core values that define Ayurveda's effectiveness and relevance in the modern healthcare landscape.

CONTINUING EDUCATION AND PROFESSIONAL DEVELOPMENT

In the dynamic field of Ayurveda, continuing education and professional development are indispensable for practitioners to stay updated, enhance their skills, and provide optimal care to their patients. Here's an exploration of their significance and impact:

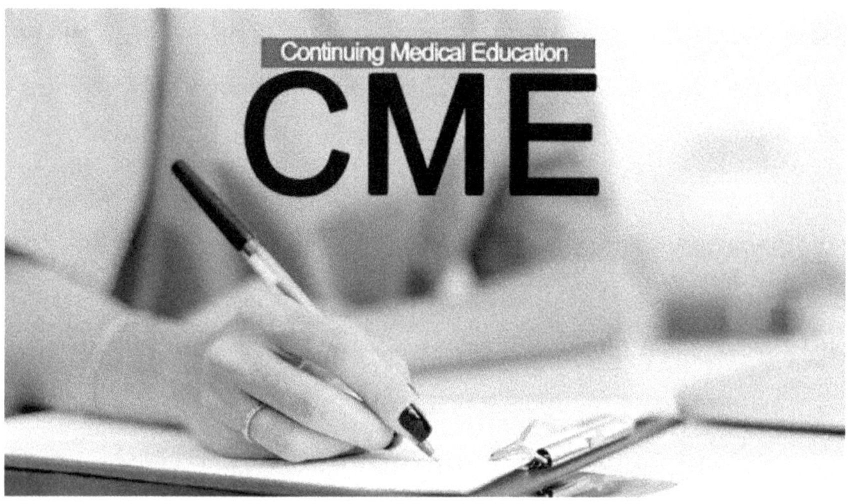

Knowledge Expansion: Continuing education offers opportunities to delve deeper into Ayurvedic principles, learn new techniques, and explore emerging research. Workshops, seminars, online courses, or advanced training programs provide access to evolving information, ensuring practitioners remain at the forefront of the field.

Skill Enhancement: Professional development allows practitioners to refine their clinical skills, deepen their understanding of specific therapies, and master diagnostic techniques. This enables them to offer more comprehensive and effective treatments tailored to individual patient needs.

Adaptation to Innovation: The landscape of healthcare constantly evolves with technological advancements and innovative practices. Continuing education equips practitioners to integrate modern tools and techniques into Ayurvedic practice while preserving the traditional wisdom that defines the discipline.

Evidence-Based Practice: Access to updated research and evidence-backed methodologies through continued education assists in aligning Ayurvedic treatments with current scientific standards. This supports evidence-based practice, enhancing credibility and acceptance within the broader healthcare community.

Professional Growth and Recognition: Ongoing education contributes to professional growth, positioning practitioners as experts in their field. Certifications, specializations, or affiliations with reputable institutions not only enhance credibility but also attract a broader patient base seeking specialized care.

Networking and Collaboration: Continuing education platforms provide avenues for networking with peers, experts, and mentors. Collaborative relationships foster knowledge exchange, opportunities for research, and potential partnerships that enrich Ayurvedic practice.

Adherence to Ethical Standards and Regulations: Education in ethical standards and legal regulations ensures practitioners maintain high ethical standards, adhere to legal frameworks, and deliver care within established guidelines, safeguarding patient trust and safety.

Personal Development: Beyond professional growth, continuing education contributes to personal development. It nurtures a practitioner's passion for Ayurveda, inspires innovation, and fosters a deeper connection to the healing art.

By embracing continuing education and professional development, Ayurvedic practitioners not only refine their skills and knowledge but also contribute to the evolution and acceptance of Ayurveda as a holistic healthcare system. It's a lifelong commitment that ensures practitioners are equipped to deliver the best possible care, making a meaningful impact on the health and well-being of their patients and the broader community.

Chapter 9

THE FUTURE OF AYURVEDA CLINICS

HIGHLIGHTS

Ayurveda's future combines ancient wisdom with modern tech, integrating personalized care and research-backed treatments, cultivating a holistic approach to wellness globally. Thriving Ayurveda clinics hinge on education, tech integration, research, and global outreach, fostering tradition alongside innovation for comprehensive healthcare.

TRENDS AND INNOVATIONS IN AYURVEDIC HEALTHCARE

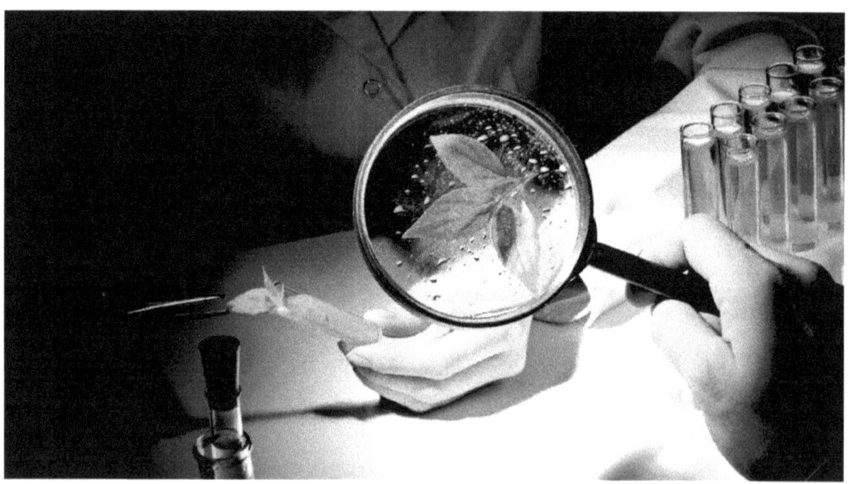

Ayurveda, a centuries-old traditional Indian system of medicine, has witnessed a resurgence in recent times due to its holistic approach to health and well-being. The convergence of modern science and technology has led to several trends and innovations in Ayurvedic healthcare.

One prominent trend is the integration of Ayurveda with conventional medicine. Many healthcare facilities now combine Ayurvedic principles with modern treatments, offering a more comprehensive approach to patient care. This integration allows for a blend of traditional remedies with evidence-based medicine, enhancing the effectiveness of treatments and broadening their acceptance.

Moreover, the digitization of Ayurvedic practices has transformed the accessibility of these ancient remedies. Mobile apps, websites, and online platforms provide information about Ayurvedic principles, herbal remedies, and personalized wellness routines. These technological advancements have made Ayurveda more accessible to a global audience, enabling people to incorporate its practices into their daily lives conveniently.

Additionally, research and development in Ayurvedic healthcare have led to innovative formulations and products. Scientific studies validating the efficacy of Ayurvedic herbs and treatments have resulted in the development of standardized herbal supplements and medicines. This fusion of traditional wisdom with modern research methodologies has expanded the range of Ayurvedic offerings and increased their credibility.

Another notable innovation is the emphasis on personalized healthcare through Ayurveda. Tailored treatment plans based on an individual's unique constitution, or "dosha," have gained popularity. This personalized approach considers a person's physical, mental, and emotional characteristics, offering customized dietary recommendations, lifestyle changes, and specific herbal formulations for optimal health outcomes.

Furthermore, the global wellness industry's growing interest in holistic healing practices has spurred the popularity of Ayurvedic therapies such as Panchakarma, herbal massages, and meditation techniques. Wellness retreats and spas offering authentic Ayurvedic experiences have become sought-after destinations for rejuvenation and relaxation.

In conclusion, the evolving landscape of Ayurvedic healthcare reflects a blend of tradition and innovation. The integration of ancient wisdom with modern science, technological advancements, personalized approaches, and product development has propelled Ayurveda to the forefront of holistic wellness practices, offering a promising path towards comprehensive healthcare.

EMBRACING TECHNOLOGICAL ADVANCEMENTS WHILE PRESERVING AYURVEDA TRADITION

The fusion of technological advancements with the ancient wisdom of Ayurveda signifies a harmonious blend that holds immense promise in revolutionizing healthcare while preserving the essence of this traditional healing system.

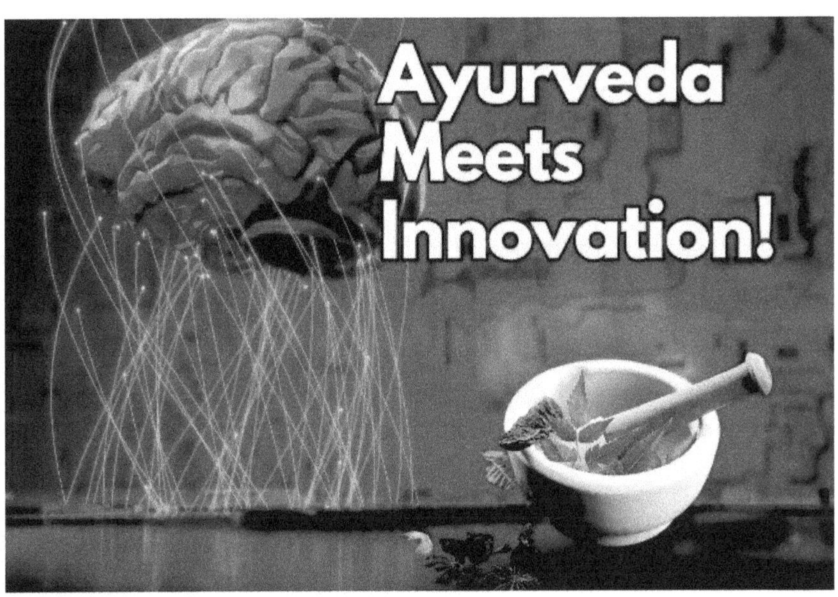

Ayurveda, a holistic healthcare system dating back thousands of years, emphasizes the balance between mind, body, and spirit for overall well-being. Its principles revolve around natural remedies, herbal formulations, personalized lifestyle modifications, and dietary practices tailored to individual constitutions.

In recent times, the integration of technology into Ayurvedic practices has amplified its reach, effectiveness, and accessibility. Digital platforms, mobile applications, and online resources have democratized access to Ayurvedic knowledge, offering guidance on remedies, lifestyle recommendations, and personalized wellness routines to a global audience.

Technological innovations have propelled Ayurveda towards greater credibility and efficiency. Research and development have facilitated scientific validation of Ayurvedic herbs and treatments, leading to the creation of standardized herbal supplements and medicines. This amalgamation of ancient wisdom with modern scientific rigor has expanded the range of Ayurvedic offerings, enhancing their efficacy and acceptance.

Moreover, the utilization of technology in Ayurvedic diagnostics and treatment has enhanced precision and personalized healthcare. Advanced diagnostic tools and techniques complement traditional methods, allowing for a more accurate assessment of an individual's constitution and health issues. This integration enables Ayurvedic practitioners to tailor treatments more effectively, aligning ancient principles with contemporary healthcare needs.

Additionally, the preservation of Ayurvedic traditions through technological means has aided in safeguarding ancient texts, knowledge, and practices. Digital libraries and repositories ensure the conservation and accessibility of centuries-old Ayurvedic texts, preserving this wealth of wisdom for future generations while making it easily accessible for scholars and practitioners worldwide.

However, while embracing technological advancements, it's crucial to maintain the authenticity and core principles of Ayurveda. Striking a balance between innovation and tradition ensures that the essence of Ayurveda's holistic healing approach remains intact.

In conclusion, the integration of technology and Ayurveda represents a harmonious synergy between ancient wisdom and modern innovation. This collaboration enhances the reach, effectiveness, and preservation of Ayurvedic practices, promising a future where traditional healing methods coexist seamlessly with cutting-edge technology, contributing to a holistic approach to health and well-being.

CULTIVATING A THRIVING FUTURE FOR AYURVEDA PRACTITIONERS

Cultivating a thriving future for Ayurveda practitioners involves several key aspects. Ayurveda, an ancient Indian holistic healing system, has gained global recognition for its emphasis on balance, natural remedies, and personalized wellness. Here are the foundational points for nurturing a prosperous future for Ayurveda practitioners:

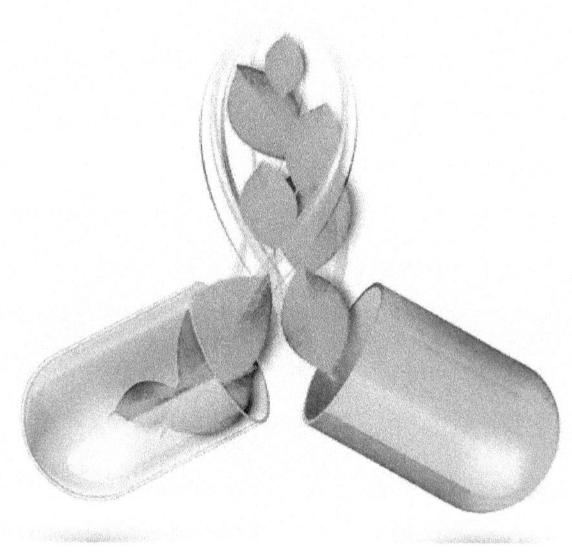

1. Education and Training

Ayurveda practitioners should have access to comprehensive, standardized, and accredited education. Continuous learning opportunities, advanced courses, and research-based training are crucial for staying updated with modern healthcare advancements while preserving Ayurvedic traditions.

2. Integration with Modern Healthcare

Collaborating with conventional healthcare systems helps Ayurveda gain broader acceptance. Integrating Ayurvedic practices with modern medicine encourages a more holistic approach to healthcare, promoting comprehensive wellness solutions.

3. Research and Development

Investing in research to validate Ayurvedic principles scientifically is pivotal. Evidence-based studies can enhance credibility, validate efficacy, and expand the application of Ayurveda in treating various health conditions.

4. Regulation and Standardization

Establishing regulatory frameworks ensures the quality, safety, and ethical practice of Ayurveda. Standardizing protocols, licensing, and certifications help build trust among practitioners and the public.

5. Global Awareness and Outreach

Increasing awareness about Ayurveda on a global scale through conferences, seminars, publications, and online platforms is essential. Building networks and alliances foster collaborations and exchange of knowledge.

6. Technological Integration

Leveraging technology for diagnosis, personalized treatment plans, and accessibility to remote patients amplifies Ayurveda's reach and effectiveness.

7. Community Engagement and Advocacy

Engaging communities to embrace Ayurveda through education, outreach programs, and advocacy initiatives creates a supportive environment for its practice.

8. Entrepreneurship and Innovation

Encouraging entrepreneurial ventures in Ayurveda, such as wellness centers, herbal product lines, and consultancy services, promotes innovation and economic growth within the field.

Conclusion

Cultivating a thriving future for Ayurveda practitioners requires a multi-faceted approach encompassing education, integration, research, regulation, global outreach, technology, community engagement, and entrepreneurial spirit. By amalgamating tradition with modernity and embracing innovation, Ayurveda can continue to evolve and positively impact healthcare globally.

RESOURCES AND REFERENCES

PROMINENT AYURVEDIC TEXTS:

Charaka Samhita: Authored by Charaka, it is one of the foundational texts of Ayurveda, focusing on general medicine and diagnosis.

Sushruta Samhita: Attributed to Sushruta, this text primarily deals with surgery, including techniques and instruments.

Ashtanga Hridaya: Written by Vagbhata, it's a concise compilation of Ayurvedic knowledge, combining Charaka and Sushruta Samhitas.

Madhava Nidanam: Focusing on diagnostics, this text is authored by Madhavakara.

Bhaishajya Ratnavali: A comprehensive work on Ayurvedic therapeutics authored by Govind Das.

Kashyapa Samhita: Attributed to Kashyapa, it emphasizes pediatrics and gynecology.

Harita Samhita: This text covers toxicology and antidotes.

Yoga Ratnakara: An Ayurvedic text that incorporates knowledge of Ayurveda and yoga practices.

Chakradatta: An ancient text that elaborates on various diseases and their treatments.

Bhavaprakasha: A comprehensive text on Ayurvedic materia medica, authored by Bhavamishra.

Sharngadhara Samhita: Another important text on Ayurvedic pharmacology, which complements the knowledge from Charaka and Sushruta Samhitas.

Nighantu Sangraha: A classic Ayurvedic text that deals with Ayurvedic pharmacology and medicinal plants.

Rasa Ratna Samuchaya: Focuses on Ayurvedic alchemy and the use of minerals and metals in medicine.

Hatha Yoga Pradipika: While not an Ayurvedic text, it contains valuable information on yogic practices and their connection to Ayurveda.

Rasendra Sara Sangraha: An important text on Rasashastra (the science of mercury and metals) and its applications in Ayurvedic medicine.

Sahasrayogam: A compendium of Ayurvedic formulations and prescriptions.

Rasa Tarangini: A classical text on Rasashastra, which deals with the preparation of metallic and mineral medicines.

Shalihotra Samhita: A text dedicated to veterinary medicine and animal care.

Agnivesha Samhita: Often considered one of the oldest texts on Ayurvedic medicine, it's the basis for the Charaka Samhita.

BOOKS BY AYUSH DEPARTMENT

The Ayush Department, part of the Indian government, has published and recommended various books and documents related to traditional Indian systems of medicine and healthcare. Some of these include:

AYURVEDIC PHARMACOPOEIA OF INDIA

NATIONAL AYURVEDIC FORMULARY OF INDIA

Publications on traditional Indian systems of medicine research, education, and practice.

The Ayush Department periodically releases and updates these documents and publications to promote and standardize the practices and medicines of Ayurveda, Yoga, Naturopathy, Unani, Siddha, and Homeopathy in India. You can find these publications on their official website or through authorized bookstores and publications.

National Ayush Morbidity and Standardized Terminologies

Standard Treatment Guidelines for Ayurveda, Siddha, and Unani

GOVERNMENT AYURVEDA ORGANISATIONS

Here are some Indian government Ayurveda organizations:

Ministry of Ayurveda, Yoga & Naturopathy, Unani, Siddha, and Homoeopathy (AYUSH)

Address: MINISTRY OF AYUSH, AYUSH BHAWAN, B Block,
GPO Complex, INA, NEW DELHI - 110023
Phone No: 011-24648354
Email: support-moayush@nic.in

Central Council for Research in Ayurvedic Sciences (CCRAS)

Jawahar Lal Nehru Bhartiya Chikitsa Avum Homeopathy
Anusandhan Bhavan
No.61-65, Institutional Area, Opp. 'D' Block, Janakpuri,
New Delhi - 110058 (India)
Telephone: 91-011-28525862/28525897/28525852

National Commission for Indian System of Medicine (NCISM)

Address: 61-65, Institutional Area, Janakpuri "D" Block,
New Delhi-110058
Email: secretary@ncismindia.org
Phone: + 91-11-28525464 / +91-11-28522519

National Institute of Ayurveda (NIA)

Jorawar Singh Gate, Amer Road

JAIPUR - 302002 (RAJ.) INDIA

Telephone: 91-141-2635816

All India Institute of Ayurveda (AIIA)

Mathura Road, Goutampuri

Sarita Vihar, Delhi 1100076

Ph: 011-26950401/402

Email: contact-us@aiia.gov.in

National Medicinal Plants Board (NMPB)

Ministry of AYUSH

Government of India

Indian Red Cross Society (IRCS),

Annexe Building, 1st & 2nd floor,1 Red Cross Road, New

Delhi-110001,

Website : www.nmpb.nic.in

Tel : 011-23721840

E-Mail ID : info-nmpb@nic.in

State Ayurvedic Colleges and Hospitals

State Ayurveda Councils and Boards

These organizations play vital roles in promoting traditional Indian systems of medicine, research, education,
and healthcare.

INDIAN AYURVEDIC ASSOCIATIONS

There are several Ayurvedic associations in India. Here are a few prominent ones:

All India Ayurvedic Congress (AIAC): AIAC is one of the oldest and most influential Ayurvedic associations in India. It promotes Ayurveda and traditional Indian medicine.

The National Integrated Medical Association (NIMA): is an Indian non-governmental organization of general practitioners educated in Ayurveda system of medicine which includes study of Modern Medicine and knowledge of ayurveda/unani/siddha with scientific approach. NIMA is officially established in 1971 with the motive to promote scientific integration of Modern Medicine & Ancient Indian Medicine i.e. ayurveda/unani/siddha.

National Ayurveda Students and Youth Association (NASYA): NASYA is a youth-oriented organization in India that focuses on promoting Ayurveda among students and young practitioners.

National Ayurvedic Medical Association (NAMA): NAMA is an organization that represents Ayurvedic professionals in India, aiming to advance the practice of Ayurveda.

Ayurveda Medical Association of India (AMAI): AMAI is an association that brings together Ayurvedic doctors and practitioners to promote Ayurvedic healthcare.

International Association for Ayurveda (IAA): While not limited to India, IAA has a presence in the country and promotes Ayurveda worldwide.

Ayurvedic Drug Manufacturers Association (ADMA): ADMA represents the interests of Ayurvedic pharmaceutical companies in India.

Ayurvedic Point of Care (APOC): APOC is a non-profit organization that focuses on Ayurvedic healthcare and research.

Association of Ayurvedic Physicians of Kerala (AAPK): AAPK is a regional association of Ayurvedic doctors in Kerala, a state known for its strong Ayurvedic tradition.

Ayurveda Pharmacy Manufacturers' Association (APMA): APMA represents the interests of Ayurvedic pharmacy manufacturers in the country.

Indian Academy of Ayurveda (IAA): IAA is dedicated to the promotion of Ayurveda through research, education, and advocacy.

Ayurvedic Graduates Medical Association (AGMA): AGMA is an association of Ayurvedic graduates who work to advance the profession and education of Ayurvedic medicine.

All India Association of Ayurvedic Graduates (AIAAG): AIAAG works to protect the rights and interests of Ayurvedic graduates and practitioners.

Indian Institute of Ayurvedic Pharmaceutical Sciences (IIAPS): IIAPS specializes in Ayurvedic pharmaceutical education and research.

Ayurveda Medical Association of India (AMAI): AMAI is another regional association representing Ayurvedic doctors and practitioners in different parts of the country.

Indian Institute of Ayurveda and Integrative Medicine (IIAIM): IIAIM is an institute that focuses on research and education in Ayurveda and integrative medicine.

Ayurveda Hospital Management Association (AHMA): AHMA is dedicated to improving the management and administration of Ayurvedic hospitals and healthcare facilities.

Ayurveda Doctors Association of India (ADAI): ADAI represents Ayurvedic doctors and practitioners across the country, advocating for the profession.

National Ayurvedic Pharmacy Association (NAPA): NAPA is an organization focused on Ayurvedic pharmacy and medication standards.

These organizations continue to play vital roles in the development and promotion of Ayurveda in India.

GLOBAL AYURVEDA ASSOCIATIONS

There are several global Ayurveda associations and organizations that promote and support the practice of Ayurveda worldwide. Some of them include:

World Ayurveda Foundation (WAF): A non-profit organization that aims to promote Ayurveda internationally and facilitate research and education in this field.

International Association of Ayurveda (IAA): A global organization that focuses on the standardization and promotion of Ayurvedic education and practice.

Ayurveda International Academy (AIA): An organization that offers Ayurveda education and certification programs to individuals and professionals worldwide.

National Ayurvedic Medical Association (NAMA): While primarily based in the United States, NAMA has members and partnerships worldwide and is dedicated to promoting Ayurveda and ensuring its integrity.

European Ayurveda Association (EUAA): Focused on promoting Ayurveda in Europe, this association connects

Ayurvedic practitioners, educators, and enthusiasts across the continent.

Ayurveda Association of Canada (AAC): This organization is dedicated to promoting Ayurveda in Canada, supporting Ayurvedic practitioners, and providing resources for those interested in Ayurveda.

Ayurveda Association of Singapore (AAOS): Focused on promoting Ayurveda in Singapore and the surrounding region, AAOS works to create awareness about Ayurveda and its benefits.

Ayurveda Association of South Africa (AASA): AASA aims to connect Ayurvedic practitioners, educators, and enthusiasts in South Africa and promote the practice of Ayurveda in the country.

Ayurveda Association of New Zealand: This organization works to support Ayurvedic practitioners, educate the public about Ayurveda, and promote the practice in New Zealand.

Ayurveda Association of Australia: Dedicated to promoting Ayurveda in Australia, this association provides information, resources, and networking opportunities for Ayurvedic practitioners and enthusiasts.

Ayurveda Practitioners' Association in the UK (APA-UK): APA-UK supports Ayurvedic practitioners in the United Kingdom and promotes Ayurveda in the region.

Ayurveda Association of Malaysia: This association focuses on Ayurveda's development and recognition in Malaysia, connecting practitioners and enthusiasts.

Ayurveda Practitioners Association of North America (APNA): APNA serves Ayurvedic practitioners and supporters in North America, facilitating networking and education.

Ayurveda Association of Latin America (AALA): AALA is dedicated to promoting Ayurveda in Latin American countries and connecting practitioners in the region.

Ayurveda Association of the Czech Republic: This organization works to establish Ayurveda in the Czech Republic and offers resources and support for practitioners and enthusiasts.

Association of Ayurvedic Professionals of North America (AAPNA): AAPNA promotes Ayurveda in North America and connects professionals and students in the field.

Ayurveda Association of Ghana: This association seeks to raise awareness of Ayurveda in Ghana and promote its practice and education.

Ayurveda Association of the Netherlands: This organization is dedicated to promoting Ayurveda in the Netherlands and connecting practitioners in the country.

Ayurveda Medical Association of India (AMAI): AMAI represents Ayurvedic medical practitioners in India and advocates for the interests of Ayurvedic doctors.

Ayurveda Practitioners' Association of Sri Lanka: This association supports Ayurvedic practitioners in Sri Lanka and works to promote traditional Ayurvedic medicine in the country.

Ayurveda Association of South Korea: Focused on Ayurveda's promotion in South Korea, this association connects Ayurvedic practitioners and enthusiasts in the country.

Ayurveda Association of the Caribbean: This organization aims to spread awareness of Ayurveda in the Caribbean region and provide resources for practitioners and individuals interested in Ayurveda.

Please keep in mind that the status and recognition of these associations may vary, and new organizations may emerge over time. It's a good practice to verify the current status and activities of these associations if you're interested in Ayurveda in specific regions.